The Calendar Book of Natural Beauty

The Calendar Book of

Drawings by Sylvia Sto

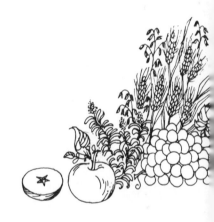

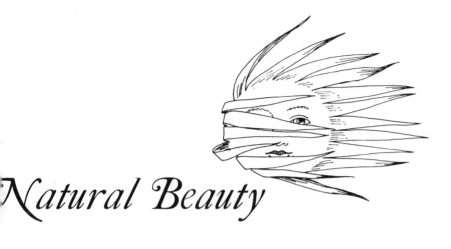

Natural Beauty

VIRGINIA CASTLETON

HARPER & ROW, PUBLISHERS
w York, Evanston
n Francisco
ndon

FIRST EDITION

Designed by Gloria Adelson

Library of Congress Cataloging in Publication Data

Castleton, Virginia.
  The calendar book of natural beauty.
  1. Beauty, Personal. I. Title.
RA778.C24   646.7'2   73-4130
ISBN 0-06-010681-6

To Mother and Ron—with gratitude and love

Contents

‎❧ᘓᘔ❧‎

Foreword

Personal beauty is a very special and highly desirable quality, for with it come great satisfaction and an incomparably warm and rewarding sense of well-being. There is certainly no woman who doesn't *want* to be beautiful, but it is up to each person to decide whether she remains just as she is or makes a real effort to improve her body, her mind, and her entire being in every way possible.

No effort toward self-improvement is ever wasted. The body always appreciates and responds to extra care, as a deprived plant opens to the sun with a flush of growth and freshness. And without the effort, life does not have that special sparkle and vitality. Because beauty, health, and spiritual satisfaction must begin within your body, it is an extravagant waste—and threat to your whole being—to ignore its daily requirements. Exercise, immaculate free-to-breathe skin, a refreshed and glowing complexion free from lines—these are the demands of a stronger, lovelier, and healthier body.

There are, undoubtedly, those women who don't make the effort needed for a good appearance, perhaps because they consider it a vain pursuit. But beauty is so closely related to health that rejecting one is very much like opposing the other. There is no more reason for you to permit early aging because of a fear of being criticized for vanity than there is a reason to allow ill health because you hesitate to pay excessive attention to your body. Since all physical beauty originates in good health, that should become your goal—and whatever leads to it should be made part of your routine.

The most attractive women in history have refused to submit passively to the imprint of time, inevitable as that may be. In actively pursuing health and beauty, they have gained many productive and enjoyable years. If there is such a thing as a natural aristocracy, it is made up of the women who use and cherish life as the exciting privilege it is and who feel the joy of living; who search for beauty in all they see and touch; and who love life and give love. To give freely and love fully, a woman must always be at her best, both spiritually and physically.

This book is intended to help women live more comfortably and contentedly by providing simple means to keep in good condition—both through good diet and old-fashioned methods, which are as modern as today's organic trend. In it I have outlined, on a month-by-month plan, a guide to natural beauty, which is the counterpart of good health. The calendar form allows you to capitalize on the richness of each season and to fall in step with nature. It is not a rigid structure but a way to know the riches— and the problems—of each season and to use the one to overcome the other.

The glow of life that comes from wholesome natural products in your diet and cosmetic regime is true beauty. And here you will learn to use the finest cosmetics—organic cosmetics. It would be senseless to suppose that though you eat nutritious food to create inner health and beauty, you use chemical, inert ingredients to feed your complexion. The integrity of the skin can be counted on only when you apply food of the finest and most nutritious sort to the body, no matter on which side.

Nature is rich with produce that supplies beauty and strength. With a living cosmetic counter everywhere around us, it taxes belief that anyone would prefer fluffy, frothy goo, with little if any value, to go on the face. A knowledgeable woman eats her oatmeal and applies a dab to her face and throat. She rubs fresh avocado onto her skin because of its rich supply of iodine, vitamin B, and vitamin A, which nourish dry skin as its oil softens and protects.

Honey and cream facials, strawberry washes for discolored skin, yeast masks for enriching natural skin tones—all these permit you to give up gels, tints, and blushes which can clog fine pores. You can stimulate hair gloss and growth with rosemary rinses and make a first-class hair conditioner from egg yolks. You can also take emerald green sprigs of mint, pungent marigold petals, crushed clusters of elderflower blossoms—all of which have been used for centuries—to create freshness, soothe distressed skin, remove wrinkles, and soften leathery complexions. Can any commercial cosmetic vie with these claims and actual feats?

These are cosmetics free for the picking, or available from a local health food store or botanical supply house (see list of supply sources). They can be easily made in your kitchen with ordinary cooking equipment. What could be simpler, healthier, or more fun?

You will shortly feel the tremendous difference between the benefits gained from using living cosmetics and those sought from the application of questionable chemical products. According to Charles Perry, English beautician and nutritionist, glycerin, boric acid, and mineral oils are only a few of the harmful ingredients in many commercial cosmetics.

Reporting on beauty aids that can damage and destroy, *Prevention* magazine quoted Dr. Eugene J. Van Scott, M.D., in a speech given at a cosmetics conference, as saying that in the past century both known and unknown carcinogenic substances have appeared in cosmetics formulas. And some, he said, are used even today.

The Nation, in its January 1, 1968, issue, reported that earlier legislation has not kept off the market hair straighteners using lye, a hair dryer with carbon tetrachloride (a potent liver poison), and a cleansing cream with "butter yellow,"—a known cancer-producing chemical. In addition, according to this report, other cosmetics, including nail polishes and shampoos that led to numerous injuries, were available to an unsuspecting public.

So turn to the natural cosmetics and experience the invigorating beauty and safety of wholesome products, of products that feed and enrich your appearance as well as enhance it.

And, of course, a healthy diet is equally essential to beauty. The menus in this book aren't meant to replace your daily diet completely, but rather to add to it, in order to assure you that you are getting the nutrients required for a well-functioning and beautiful body. Because a wholesome and nutritious diet is so very important to beauty and health, a meal should not just happen, but should be carefully planned to include those nutrients which may be in short supply in the body because of a casual attitude toward food and the availability of "quickie" meals, which rob you of vitality and life.

Both the breakfasts and lunches listed are easy to prepare, and offer a wealth of food value. The dinners are uncomplicated and delicious, stressing many unusual foods that are rich in energy-giving nutrients and low in calories.*

Little beef is used. Americans generally rely too much on the muscle meats of beef, pork, and the like for protein sources. To counter this and to offer variety, I have substituted other delicious protein foods. You could try two or three of the menus a week, and see whether your meals aren't more interesting and your body lighter. For the menus given in each month are truly beauty bringers in their wholesome deliciousness. Bon appetit!

So begin at the beginning or borrow from any month you choose to add to another month's benefits. In fact, this book could be considered a primer in that you won't forget what you learned on page one merely because you reach page five. Instead, garner all its bits of knowledge and add them to your fullness of days. And at the end of the book, or year, you will have built a body of beauty practices that, duly performed, have made you into the attractive and serene woman you were intended to be.

---

* In each chapter, recipes are provided for those starred dishes in the monthly menus.

After bringing out her best, a woman can turn with poise and confidence to the areas of interest she feels committed to. No longer will she struggle with self-doubt and displeasure about the condition of her body. It really takes very little time to bring out your best through extra care, and once you have formed the habit, it becomes second nature. We have been given time to use it well, and those who think they don't have enough to be at their best should remember that time is a form of love, and that, by stinting on one, the other can be lost.

Virginia Castleton

Editor's Note

Not every person responds to every cosmetic substance in exactly the same way and, even with totally natural substances such as those given in this book, there may occasionally be the possibility of an allergic reaction. So please apply the recipes and formulas with care. If you have any doubt about a particular ingredient or compound, try a small amount first to make sure that you are not unusually sensitive to it.

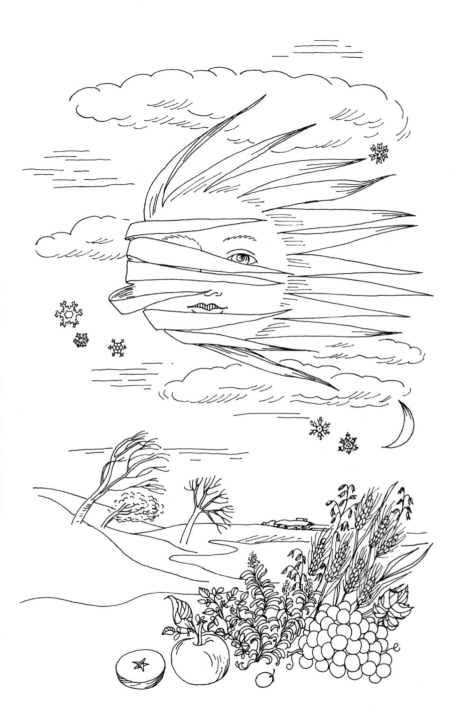

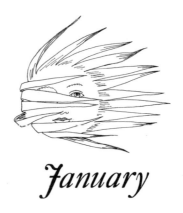

January

Come, cold winds, at January's call,
On whistling wings, and with white
flakes bestrew
The earth.

    John Ruskin: "The Months"

This is the month that was dedicated to Janus, the god of two faces who could look into both the departed year and the one before him. Called Frosty Month by the Dutch, January was referred to by the Saxons as Wolf Month because the scarcity of food brought the wolves nearer and nearer their habitations. On the French revolutionary calendar, it was known as Snow Month.

January remains, of course, a month of cold winds, and of snow, and dry desert winds in those areas. For those who are cold-weather people with a love for sporting on ski slopes and crystallized lakes, preparation and after care must be given the face and body to prevent winter damage to delicate skin tissue.

Pamper and nourish the winter body with a satiny oatmeal bath, a creamy food facial, and gentle exercises which revitalize, restore, and return to you a figure which is beautifully your own.

And look toward tomorrow, as Janus did.

OATMEAL BATH FOR JANUARY

Cold-weather beauty bathing can yield almost immediate results, especially if done with oatmeal. Oatmeal, I sometimes think, is the wonder treatment of them all. It is one of the richest known beauty foods and is highly rewarding both in the diet and for external use on the body. Its high mineral content of potassium and phosphorus, calcium and magnesium makes it a valuable food source. In addition, its high vitamin B content, along with some vitamin E and G, increases its cosmetic value.

In accordance with our belief that what is good for the body internally will also profit you externally, stepping into the opulence of an oatmeal bath is an open invitation to the body to soak up these rich nutrients. Softening, bleaching, and just plain pampering are some of the benefits to be gained from an oatmeal bath.

With winter winds denuding one's scant skin oils, and heated rooms further destroying natural skin health, frequent oatmeal baths in the winter months give the body a chance to recuperate, to ward off the disadvantages of modern living, and to provide a protective screen for the skin tissue.

Oatmeal Beauty Bath

1 cup old-fashioned oatmeal   2 cups water

Grind 1 cup of the dry oats in a blender or nut grinder. Reduce to a powder and mix with 2 cups of warm water by adding the water to the oatmeal in the blender. After thoroughly mixing, add 2 additional cups of warm water and continue to blend.

Strain the milky fluid through gauze. Pour the liquid into your tub of bath water, filled no more than half full for the best effects. Then catch up the corners of the gauze and knot them into a bagful of the oatmeal. Drop the bag into the tub to gain the full benefits of the oatmeal and also use it as a washcloth.

Take this bath daily for the entire month of January, without using soap on your body, and without any rinsing other than with the water in the tub.

DRY HAIR OIL PACK

Beautiful hair is a great asset, but its maintenance can be a source of unhappiness because of today's harsh detergent shampoos, insufficient vegetable oils in the diet, and reluctance to use the hairbrush properly and daily. One problem in particular—dry hair—plagues a large percentage of women. It can be overcome to a great degree by switching to an herbal, egg, or castile shampoo, and using a dry hair oil pack.

Brush the hair thoroughly, covering every area of the scalp and hair itself. Bend forward from the waist and begin stroking in long movements from the very edge of the back of the scalp all the way to the front in one continuous movement with the brush. This thorough cleansing will remove all loose dandruff, which usually accompanies dry hair, and stimulate the scalp for the warm oil treatment to follow.

Heat a generous amount of sesame seed, safflower, olive, or other nut or vegetable oil in a custard cup placed in a pan of hot water. Massage the oil into the scalp from back to front, covering every area. Continue to massage through the hair until every strand is saturated, then draw a comb gently through the hair several times to distribute the oil better.

Dip an absorbent towel into hot water and wring it out a

bit. Wrap the towel turban-style around the head and fasten it tightly to keep in the heat. Sit under your hair dryer if you have one. If not, wind clear plastic around the toweling to keep the heat in as long as possible. (Do not use the plastic if you sit under the dryer.)

As the towel cools, remove it and dip it again into hot water and rewrap it around the head. Thirty minutes of this should do wonders for your dry hair. Remove excess oil by shampooing thoroughly with an herbal shampoo. Thick hair may require two shampoos. Use a tablespoon of apple cider rinse in the last rinse water, or that amount of lemon juice for light hair.

In France, corrective shampoos for all types of hair are available. Many of them are prepared from a lanolin base which is excellent for damaged, dry hair. Repeated shampooing with these products seems to saturate the badly damaged hair follicles and coat them with the lamb's wool fat that is so easily absorbed by the human body, because of all animal fats, it is the most similar to that of the human body. These superfatted strands are then able to withstand frequent shampooing and setting to a degree not possible before. Other shampoos on the market there include wild herb mixtures which leave the hair clean and treated with nature's own healing products.

Of course, there are just as many modern products on the commercial market in France as in any other country. But many French women have never given up homier concoctions which incorporate every known beneficial plant and vine.

Herbal shampoos usually have a castile soap base to which one or a variety of herbs is added, depending on the hair qualities you wish to achieve. Easily available today in health food shops, mail-order houses, and even in drug and department stores, these shampoos are generally safe for problem hair and are very effective cleansers for most hair types.

If you would like to experiment on your own, you could start with ½ teaspoon of lanolin beaten into 1 teaspoon of polyunsaturated oil and 1 tablespoon of water, mixed together over boiling water. This is then beaten into 2 tablespoons of herbal shampoo. If the shampoo proves too soapy, next time add a bit more lanolin and oil, in minute proportions.

This shampoo will give a beautiful gloss to the hair, and additional body because it coats the hair shafts. Use apple cider or lemon rinse afterward, to remove any excess oil and soap.

OILY HAIR

Brushing is essential with oily hair, just as it is with dry hair. The bristles lift and distribute the oil to the outer ends of the hair with this action, helping to lessen the heavy concentration of oil around the roots which clogs the fine pore openings.

An excellent means of ridding hair of its oily excess is to use a gauze stretched over the bristles in the brush. This will catch the dust and oily wastes and remove them, while pulling up the heavier flow of oil around the roots and stimulating the scalp at the same time.

A good shampoo for oily hair will cleanse both scalp and hair and yet not strip the hair of all essential oils; this can be found in some herbal or castile shampoos. Sometimes the overactive sebaceous glands are stimulated by too-frequent shampoos. It is important to correct this fault from within, by improving nutrition. Thus, substitute polyunsaturated fats for animal fats in the diet, in addition to other good nutritional practices. Fatty and fried foods should be eliminated from the diet as well as pastries, alcohol, and too many starches.

A rosemary hair rinse is considered infallible in helping to eliminate oily hair. Antiseptic and valuable as a tonic, rosemary rinse has been used for centuries by women with problem hair. In addition to helping control oily scalp and hair, this herbal solution helps eliminate hair loss while strengthening and brightening the hair.

One of the greatest investments anyone with oily or thin hair can make is the purchase and preparation of this herbal liquid. Rosemary leaves can be ordered from botanical supply houses or purchased from health food stores or herbalists shops. It would be more reasonable to buy rosemary in those places than in a supermarket, where it is sold as a seasoning.

A 3½ ounce box, costing less than a dollar, will provide nearly two dozen applications.

Rinse for Oily Hair

½ cup dried rosemary leaves   2 cups cold water

Place the herbs in a glass, steel, or enamel pot and pour the cold water over them. Heat over the lowest flame possible for 10 minutes or until the boiling point is reached. Maintain a low simmering temperature for 5 minutes before removing the pot from the heat. Allow the brew to steep overnight, with a lid on the pot. Next morning, pour the mixture into a clean jar and pour off the amount needed each day.

Rub enough of the herbal liquid into the scalp nightly to cover the scalp and hair roots completely. Even greater benefits come from lightly massaging the rosemary rinse throughout the hair and scalp, wetting all the strands of hair. Continue to massage the scalp and fluff the hair for quicker drying.

Facial Cleanser for an Oily Skin

It isn't always a good idea to wash the face repeatedly with water and soap. According to the time of year, there can be a more than desirable loss of facial oils. Instead of using plain water, try instead a meaningful facial cleanser such as a vegetable or fruit. Not only will these cleanse, but there is a nourishing element included as a bonus.

The common but wonderful potato can be added to your beauty regimen with splendid results. Rich in vitamins B, C, and G, and a good source of sulfur, the potato can clear oily skin while adding softening qualities if used often enough.

Cut a slice from an Irish potato. With a serrated knife, crisscross the potato until it becomes somewhat pulpy. Rub this gently onto every area of the face and allow the liquid to dry 15 to 20 minutes before rinsing away, without soap, and patting dry.

DRY SKIN

Rub a slice of apple, whose surface has been scratched to make it soft, across the dry complexion and leave it on for thirty minutes before rinsing away without using soap. Apply a thin coating of vegetable or nut oil and blot dry.

JANUARY HAND SHIELD

Preventing chapped hands should begin with the first raw winds and continue right through the first soft breezes. January's chilling winds bite into unprotected hands, and even wearing gloves is not always a guarantee that you will escape the unattractive reddened skin that suggests negligence and discomfort. If you are careless in drying your hands or if you don't apply really effective protective creams or lotions as a shield, the thin skin on the backs of your hands will usually redden upon exposure.

In earlier days, women who were really concerned with their hands often wore two pairs of gloves—considered even better insulators than one thick pair. To avoid that bother, try using a little sweet almond or sesame seed oil lotion.

Prepare this by thoroughly shaking together ½ teaspoon of the oil, 1 teaspoon fresh lemon juice or apple cider vinegar, and ¼ teaspoon of honey. Blend well each time before using. Rub into your hands, then hold them briefly under warm running water. Pat dry with soft paper toweling, and you will then have left on your hands a thin protective film of softening and shielding nutrients which is not oily or sticky but which does so much more for your hands than the usual insipid lotion.

TIRED SKIN

With the holidays over and the extravagant dining that usually accompanies them a guilty memory, it is time to take stock of your appearance and set to work to correct the results of any dietary extravagance.

The quantities of sweets and alcohol consumed during the holidays is bound to show on your face and body. As a matter of fact, within minutes of consuming alcohol, the skin on a woman's face will slacken noticeably. Dull, lifeless skin can also result from prolonged exposure to harsh winds and other winter assaults. A revivifying facial can do a great deal toward restoring a lost complexion, especially if nutrition habits are improved at the same time.

A rich cream facial using ingredients from the kitchen can practically lift the wrinkling caused by dry skin and smooth the skin back to its former lineless beauty. Used daily and allowed to remain on the skin for at least 15 minutes—though preferably 30 minutes—the thick cream base with its added collagenous protein both feeds and sustains the tissue, and coaxes softness back to the offended skin.

Food Cream for Tired Skin

1 fertile egg, available at
    health food stores
2 tablespoons apple cider
    vinegar

½ teaspoon sea salt
1 cup cold processed salad
    oil

Place the egg, apple cider vinegar, salt, and half of the oil into a blender and cover. Blend at a high speed until the mixture thickens. Remove the cover of the blender and pour a steady but very slow stream of the remaining oil into the blender while it continues to run at a high speed. Blend together thoroughly. If necessary, stop the blender and scrape the sides down and rerun until homogenized. This is the basic cream.

Make only half of the cream base at a time into the final cosmetic. Add 2 tablespoons of collagenous protein to ½ cup of the cream base. (Collagenous protein can be bought at a health food store or beauty shop.) Add 2 tablespoons of oatmeal water (see below) and beat together well. Keep refrigerated until needed.

For best results, apply the facial cream to a clean face and gently massage it into all areas of the face and throat every day for a month.

Oatmeal Water

Soak 2 tablespoons of oatmeal in 6 tablespoons of hot water for 5 minutes. Strain through gauze and add 2 tablespoons of this milky fluid to the cream base and collagenous protein.

WINTER TAN

Turn your back on winter and its pallor and absolutely glow with make-believe tan, if you prefer the bronze to the Camille look. And it is cheering to see something this month that suggests sunshine and warmer days. While this homemade sunshine lotion won't actually tan your skin, it will give it a lovely deepened shade and at the same time add its own super softness from its lanolin base.

This formula was devised by a model who couldn't afford a trip south but who refused to be a pale goddess in February and who had a knowledge of homemade cosmetics. And now, with the growing knowledge of skin damage which results from overexposure to the sun's rays, many of her friends are deserting harsh sun baths for this formula tan.

Cook (yes, cook) over very low heat 2 tea bags in half a cup of water for 15 minutes, mashing the bags from time to time to extract the full color strength from the tea. Salvage a quarter cup of this darkened brew and set aside.

Set a largish glass custard cup over hot water and melt 2 tablespoons each of lanolin and sesame seed oil. Remove from the heat and very slowly, just as in making mayonnaise, pour in the tea, almost drop by drop, beating all the while. Continue beating until the mixture is homogenized. Massage into the areas where you want a suntan and luxuriate in your winter color.

CHAPPED-HAND BALL

If you've failed to use your hand-shielding lotion each time before you go out or if you've acquired roughened, reddened hands from indoor work, then it is time for heroic measures to bring your hands back to an attractive state. Nothing seems to heal them faster than the old-fashioned and, today, little-practiced use of camphor in a soothing wax base.

Our great grandmothers, who sometimes had almost unbearable tasks to perform with no help from labor-saving devices and protective rubber gloves, found this formula totally effective for combating chafed hands.

Melt 3 teaspoons of spermaceti and 4 teaspoons of white beeswax. Add 1 ounce of almond oil. Moisten 3 teaspoons of camphor with enough brandy to make a paste and blend all together. Pour into molds. (Bottle lids will do and so will egg cups; use whatever gives the shape you want your hand ball to take. Or, roll into balls by molding the warm mixture between the palms of your hands.)

Rub the ball gently across your hands and palms, covering both the inside and outside.

HERBAL STEAM FACIAL

Moisture is sapped from the exposed skin during the winter months, and by exposure to drying winds in warmer parts of the country. Dry, flaking skin can result from these extremes of temperature. One of the quickest ways to a new skin appearance is with the use of a facial herb steaming. This very effective application can actually remove the dead top layer of skin and release the newer underskin, permitting it to come forth with a smoother, porcelain-like texture. Only then will the application of oils and creams for softer skin become truly effective. But directions must be followed carefully or this method of restoration simply does not work.

Time is of great importance in the facial herb steaming. Apparently it is effective only if used for the full fifteen minutes recommended. Do not use for a longer or shorter period of time.

The facial steam is an application of hot, moist cloths which have been dipped into a fragrant herbal mixture and held against the face, covering it completely. As the cloth loses its heat and cools, it is removed, dipped once again into the herbal mixture, squeezed slightly, and placed against the face again.

To prepare the solution, drop 2 papaya mint tea bags into 2 cups of boiling water. Simmer 3 or 4 minutes, remove from the heat, and use while quite warm. Time should not be lost between applications, as it is the continual heat and herbal mixture which successfully loosen the dead scarf skin debris.

You might be more comfortable lying down as you apply the cloths, and in that way you won't be forced to hold them in place with your hands. However, the bother of jumping up and down to change the cloths every two or three minutes makes some women prefer to stand. Turn on the radio and listen to music, practice your French, do mental gymnastics, or whatever you choose. But do use your mind during this tedious but highly successful beauty treatment.

After 15 minutes, splash cool, not cold, water on the face. Apply a thin film of nut or fruit oil to the face and blot. Your skin will be rosy, and remain so for a while. Never use this formula just before going out. At night, just before retiring, is the best time to use the facial. By morning, the deep flush is gone and you are left with a new, glowing skin, fresh to the touch and free to breathe.

If you have broken facial veins, don't use the hot compresses. Instead, mash a very ripe papaya and spread it on the face. Allow it to remain for 30 minutes and rinse with warm water. Rub the skin gently with a towel, removing the loosened surface tissue. Rinse again in warm and then in cool water.

POMANDER FOR JANUARY

During January pomanders for scenting can brighten your day, lift your mind, and assault your heart with nostalgia. Their historic heritage brings to mind the days of extravagance when tiny Spanish oranges were stuck with cloves and other spices or herbs and worn suspended from a lady's girdle, like some ornament.

Pomanders were the creation of fanciful imaginations, and they ranged from the beautifully simple orange to carefully wrought gold and silver reproductions of the fruit. But no one has improved on the exquisitely scented fruit pomanders.

Choose a perfect orange, lemon, or lime. Stick the pointed end of the cloves into the skin to form a close pattern marching up and down and around the fruit, with one clove top touching the next. Dry the fruit in a cool area for a month. Then prepare a mixture of equal amounts of powdered orris root, cinnamon, nutmeg, allspice, and cloves. Roll the fruit in this powdered mixture until it is well coated, then enclose with the remaining powder in a closed container for a week.

Remove the fruit from the box and shake free of the loose powder. Tie the by-now beautifully scented pomander with two ribbons, creating quarter sections, and tie the tops to form a loop. Use in your closet, bedroom, bathroom, or any place you wish to scent.

APHRODISIAC FOR JANUARY

According to the ancient Greeks, Aphrodite, goddess of love and beauty, has ruled women and men from the earliest days of existence. And it was among the Greeks that certain foods, wines, herbs, and flowers became endowed with sensuous powers and were associated with success in love.

Philters of suggestion, excitement, and seduction were created from a wild variety of ingredients, some of them indigestible and some parts of a regular menu—not because they were especially successful, but because they tasted so good.

But the interest in promoting romance through the use of stimulants has continued down to our own blasé age. Do we not serve wine with candlelit dinners when we feel romantic? And men now swallow vitamin E capsules for virility much as a Grecian lover might have consumed honey cakes for increased sexual prowess or the object of his love might have had mint tea to make her respond more readily.

As to what constitutes an aphrodisiac, no one really seems certain. Foods highest on the list of aphrodisiacs generally seem to contain a larger amount of minerals than others. There are a couple of items which are powerful sexual stimulants, but they are considered harmful and are generally unobtainable. We'll concentrate, therefore, on our own brand of aphrodisiacs, which are a sensuous delight to the taste even if they may not necessarily turn you on sexually.

We believe that aphrodisiacs are largely cerebral, anyway. But for fun—and possible profit—try the aphrodisiac of the month. It will, in any event, be a taste treat, besides making you healthier. And maybe that is just the aphrodisiac we all need.

Honey of Heaven

¾ cup almond meal
2 cups milk
2 egg yolks
¼ teaspoon nutmeg

¾ cup honey
1 tablespoon arrowroot
Extra milk, as needed

Blend together the almond meal, milk, egg yolks, and nutmeg. Heat the honey until it bubbles, and slowly beat into the first mixture. Dissolve the arrowroot in enough additional cold milk to make a thin paste and stir into the first mixture. Blend well, place over a low flame, and stir until it thickens. Serve the drink warm.

EXERCISES FOR A SUPPLE BACK

The condition of the back can reveal an aged appearance as easily as the face. When the spine ceases to be limber, physical movement slows up, leading to stiff posture, rounded shoulders, a thickened waistline, and other undesirable consequences. Surplus flesh begins to accumulate around the shoulders, rolls of unattractive flesh spread around confining undergarments, and the overblown middle-aged look intensifies, no matter how youthful the face.

When muscles slacken and grow weak, skin folds begin to appear. In order to avoid this condition, exercises should begin early in life. However, if you have neglected your body and find yourself in the middle years with damage already in evidence, there is still a chance to resurrect your appearance and grow younger in both body and fact.

Think of the vertebrae as the support of your body and you

will always stand tall and maintain good posture. To find that outline and to learn the condition of your spine, try the back-check test.

Stand straight with your back pressed against the wall. Place the feet together with the knees slightly bent. Slowly start pressing your spine to the wall, beginning at the lowest part. Allow your knees to straighten as your back presses backward.

In the beginning, it is not likely that your entire back will touch the wall. But continued practice eventually makes this possible. This straightened position will help eliminate the ungainly swayback look brought about by poor posture.

To limber the spine further, sit on the floor in loose clothing. Make a ball of your body by bringing the knees up and under the chin and closing your arms around the knees from the side. Drop your head to your knees and slowly rock backward in a rounded position. Without stopping, rock forward again. Repeat this rocking-ball position several times.

Continued practice will help create flexibility in the stiffened vertebrae, and bring on a youthfulness of movement and a toning to the body. In addition, body tension will begin to disappear, for in flexing the entire vertebrae length, the neck muscles ease. And since it is in this area that tension begins to build up, this exercise serves many purposes of beauty by adding relaxation and serenity to a rigid body.

BREAKFASTS FOR JANUARY

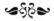

Prunes cooked with honey
Whole-grain oatmeal with raisins
Herbal tea

Cranberry juice
Poached egg
Whole wheat toast
Sunflower meal and honey spread*
Herbal tea

Bowl of sliced oranges
Granola*
Herbal tea

Stewed apricots
Brown rice flour pancakes*
Herbal tea

Bananas in milk
Egg and onion omelet
Cornmeal chapaties with sunflower meal and honey spread*
Herbal tea

Stewed apples
Oatmeal with currants
Herbal tea

Grape juice
Brown rice and raisins
Herbal tea

LUNCHES FOR JANUARY

⋙

Broth made of chicken stock and onions
Bowl of grated carrots, beets, and green peppers with ground
  sesame seed meal
Yogurt

Bouillon with whole wheat crackers and cream cheese
Salad of shredded cabbage, beets, celery, and turnips
Yogurt

Barley soup
Zucchini, radish, and grated carrot salad with cheese
Yogurt

Chicken broth
Brown rice salad*
Yogurt with sliced banana

Pumpkin soup (recipe on p. 263)
Cheese and fruit
Yogurt

Cabbage soup
Apple slices spread with peanut butter
Whole wheat sandwich of ground sunflower meal and honey spread*
Yogurt

Whole potato soup*
Watercress and orange salad
Yogurt

DINNERS FOR JANUARY

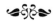

Braised liver
Steamed broccoli with lemon and oil
Sweet potatoes

Lentil bean loaf*
Turnips with oil and herbal seasoning
Mustard greens

Cheese soufflé
Brussels sprouts
Stewed tomatoes

Braised sweetbreads
Whole mashed potato
Coleslaw

Baked acorn squash and cheese
String beans
Cornmeal chapaties*

Lean ground meat patties of ½ heart and ½ beef
Potato pancakes (recipe on p. 238)
Wilted spinach and onion

Chicken and brown rice casserole
Broccoli

RECIPES FOR JANUARY

Sunflower Meal and Honey Spread

Grind a handful of hulled sunflower seeds and mix with enough honey to make a soft paste. Keep refrigerated.

Granola

¼ cup dates, chopped	1 cup soy flour
½ cup water	1 cup corn meal
1 cup honey	1 cup nutmeats
¾ cup salad oil	1 cup grated coconut
2 cups rolled oats	¼ cup dried apricots
2 cups whole wheat flour	1 teaspoon salt

Mix the dates and water in blender and add honey and oil to this mixture. Pour into bowl containing all the other ingredients and mix until it all has a crumbly texture. Spread out onto a large, flat pan and roast in oven at 275 degrees until golden in color.

Brown Rice Flour Pancakes

1 egg	1 cup self-rising brown rice flour
1¼ cups milk	¼ tablespoon salad oil

Beat egg and add milk. Stir in the flour and beat smooth. Add the oil and allow to rest for 10 minutes. Bake on a hot griddle.

Brown Rice Salad

2 tomatoes
1 green pepper
1 cup cooked brown rice
¼ teaspoon salt

2 tablespoons salad oil
1 tablespoon lemon juice
dill

Chop tomatoes and green pepper and stir into rice. In a separate container, mix together the oil, lemon juice, salt, and dill, or other seasoning such as sweet basil, savory, etc. Pour over the rice and vegetable mixture and allow to season for 1 hour.

Whole Potato Soup

Cut one whole potato with the skin on, into cubes and cook in chicken broth or bouillon. Puree while hot in the blender and add milk until the consistency is soupy. Season to taste.

Lentil Bean Loaf

2 cups cooked lentils
½ cup whole wheat crumbs
½ cup chopped pecans
½ teaspoon summer savory
1 teaspoon salt

1 chopped onion
4 tablespoons salad oil
¾ cup milk
1 egg

Mash lentils with a potato masher to a crumbly consistency. Blend in all the dry ingredients and the onion. Add the oil and milk to the beaten egg, combine with lentil mixture, form a loaf, and place on an oiled flat pan. Bake at 350 degrees for 1 hour. Serve with a tomato sauce seasoned with lemon juice.

Cornmeal Chapaties

¾ cup finely ground corn-
    meal
½ teaspoon baking powder

1 teaspoon sea salt
1 beaten egg
1½ cups milk

Combine egg and milk and pour into dry ingredients, blending until smooth. Bake on hot greased griddle until bubbles form. Turn and brown on the other side.

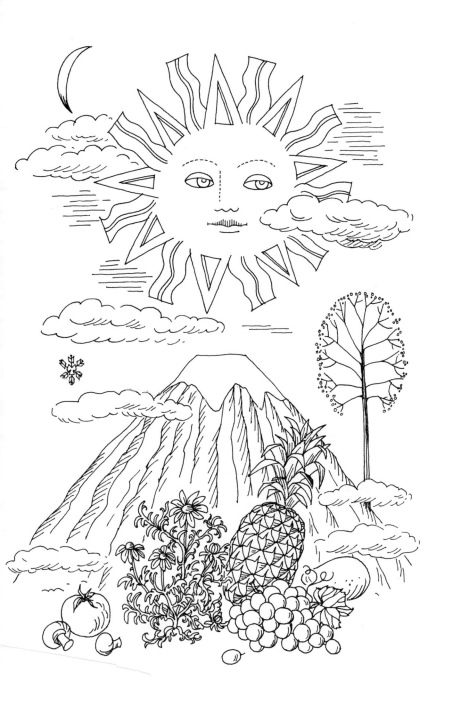

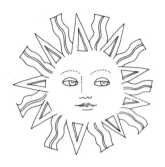

February

Come when the rains have glazed the
snows
And clothed the trees with ice,
While the slant sun of February pours
Into the bowers a flood of light.

William Cullen Bryant:
"A Winter Place"

This was the month of purification for the Romans, and the Anglo-Saxons called it "sprout kale," referring to cabbage or kale, one of the first green things to grow. In the French Republic calendar, it was called Rain Month.

And so it remains, this rainy, cold month during which the earth is soaked in preparation for the coming growth. And we in turn must acknowledge the cold and the damp and realize that we cannot hibernate in cozy comfort without care but, rather, must daily provide for and sustain our winter bodies through winter's worst.

Your body can really be abused by February's unkind weather if you don't maintain careful watch and practice preventive beauty care. Good skin care seems to fall into three phases, each essential to the other. You must first cleanse the skin, then feed it, and finally protect it. No one practice can take the place of any other, and the three together can indeed bring gratifying results.

Preventive beauty care suggests elimination of most soaps, especially during the colder months, for their alkaline addition to the skin merely succeeds in increasing its dryness and rough texture. For cleansing the skin, use a lovely cream oil mixture that helps avoid the use of water on sensitive skins and at the same time does a splendid job of removing makeup.

Feeding the needy complexion with a honey-egg facial nourishes and softens it, bringing a double benefit in its rich nutrients. Then try an oil bath that soothes and smooths itchy drying skin, and strike out at February's cruel weather. According to tacticians, the best defense is a good offense. Following through on that bit of strategy, use a protective hand cream that will help you avoid chapped red hands. And if you've not done your homework in preventive plotting, don't worry, velveteen cream for chafed hands will quickly improve the situation.

During these sunless months, you can also ward off the grayness of cloudy skies that seek to dull your complexion by using a tingling earth stimulator for creating pink-hued cheeks. Causing no more bother than a thirty-minute nap or resting period (absolutely essential to your best appearance), a Fuller's Earth facial can wreathe you in a pastel glow you couldn't get outside of Key Largo or the top of a Swiss mountain after a day's skiing.

There are other benefits in February's busy calendar. Bathe the hair lovingly and rewardingly in a super cleansing shampoo of fresh eggs which is a companion formula to the egg facial. Both hair and skin will thirstily absorb the protein of this basis-of-life food.

Or massage in the astringent qualities coming from the American witch hazel shrub and save yourself an extra shampoo, hoarding the needed oils for dry hair rather than depleting them.

And don't forget that while every month, week, and day should have you practicing good eye care, good vision can become especially strained during the months with little or no sun. Check your intake of vitamin D, the sunshine vitamin, and add additional strength to strained eyes by practicing some mild exercises. This is as much a part of regular beauty care as the protection and improvement of any other part of the body.

So, feed the body this month with all kinds of little extras, and watch it glide through February. The slant sun of February will seem but a moment's duration when you see the improvement in your entire body.

BEAUTY GRAINS FOR FEBRUARY

Winter brings a host of skin problems to the unwary. Many of these difficulties can be traced to a lack of fresh fruits and vegetables, to convenience meals that have no sustaining life and therefore cannot impart the glow that comes from good nutrition. In consequence, a starving skin can rebel in many ways. The peeling, flaky winter gray look that hits around this time of year can many times be traced to a nutritional deficiency.

Whatever the cause—faulty diet or staying too long indoors in overheated and drying temperatures—correct it and then attack your flaky skin. A more than adequate means of doing this is with the use of plain iodized salt or sea salt. Dissolve 1 teaspoon of salt in enough water to fill a small spray bottle. Keeping the eyes closed and avoiding the area directly beneath them, spray the salt water solution right onto both face and neck. Allow this to dry and begin rubbing gently at the skin, treating it very gently but creating enough friction to loosen and remove the cellular waste. Beneath the useless top surface, once it is removed, the complexion should be glowing fresh and pink. Rinse well several times and apply a soothing film of oil or cream.

EXERCISES

In winter, when you are confined indoors more than you'd like to be and should be, exercise means a great deal. Improvement in carriage, complexion, and clearness of vision can come from an exercise that relaxes the body even as it strengthens the neck muscles and brings an added blood supply to the upper part of the body. Rotate your head slowly to limber the part of the body that can become a collection point for tension and irritation. By flexing the neck muscles, stiffness is relieved and the blood is allowed to circulate more easily.

Stand tall with your head centered between your shoulders. Drop your head, without moving your shoulders, toward your chest, with your chin as close to your chest as is comfortably possible. This will stretch the spinal column forward and you doubtlessly will hear the creaking sounds of decalcified and under-exercised bones. Do not strain or force your neck to move in a wider circle than it easily can.

In slow motion, roll your head in a complete circle around to the left and backward and on around to the right. Slowly, but without stopping, continue to roll your head. Remember to hold your shoulders still, moving only your head. Reverse the position and swing slowly in the opposite direction. Two or three rounds of this exercise is sufficient the first few days. Gradually increase the rolls as your neck muscles develop more ease.

OIL BATH FOR FEBRUARY

Depleted oil supplies will lead this month to the discomfort of itching, scaly skin which in no way resembles your skin of warmer months. With scratchy winter clothing rubbing against achingly dry skin, you can end up with a sandpapery texture which is both uncomfortable and unkind.

To hold on to the supple skin of good health and youth requires patience and consideration. The skin you love to touch and to have touched and yearn to maintain will fast slip away if you are a quick-shower type and never indulge in a luxurious and meaningful bath.

Only if you cherish your body and consider its many needs can you continue year after year as a woman of beauty who is remembered for her charm of appearance. Treat your body as tenderly as you would a child's. Cleanse it gently, oil it lavishly, and feed it daily. Rub in quantities of healing caressing lotions and oils. In February, counter the bleakness of sunless days and skin-drying conditions by pouring your own skin conditioner into the bathwater. In addition to your daily vitamin D supplements, let your body soak in the soft, satiny splendor of an oil-rich bath.

Avoid the use of regular toilet soaps during the harsher winter months. Soap really isn't necessary if you replace it with other cleansers like herbal baths, salt rubs, and oatmeal and bran bag washcloths. These delightful preparations will lift the debris from your skin far more effectively than soap, which merely cleanses the top surface and leaves its own deposit.

Use this February bath to make your skin feel as supple as it was ten or twenty years ago.

Oil Bath

1 cup sweet almond oil
1 tablespoon of herbal
    shampoo

½ teaspoon oil of rosemary

Blend all ingredients with an egg beater or by placing in the blender and going from the slowest to the highest speed. Start running your bathwater and then pour 4 tablespoons of this mixture directly beneath the hot water faucet, allowing the force of the water to homogenize the oil into the bath. Do not use soap, but soak in this revitalizing brew for 15 to 20 minutes before toweling the skin vigorously.

EYE CARE

In the winter we are indoors too much—and we suffer the consequences. Cigarette smoke in the office burning your eyes? Too many parties? Clear your strained vision by bathing your eyes in a refreshing herbal solution.

Mix equal parts of chamomile, fennel, and eyebright herbs to make 1 heaping teaspoonful. Pour a cup of boiling water over the herbs and allow them to steep for 5 minutes. Strain. When just barely warm, dip sterilized cotton into the infusion and bathe the eyes repeatedly.

You can carry a small bottle of this herbal solution to the office and use it daily for soothing eyes fatigued by paper work, stale air, or even lack of sleep.

Fennel is an aromatic member of the parsley family, noted for its iron content. Inflamed eyes benefit from a solution made of the fennel seeds. Chamomile adds a tonic freshness to an eye solution, and eyebright has long been recognized as a valuable astringent in such preparations. According to the medieval doctrine of signatures, which asserts that a plant's use can be found on stalk, stem, flower, or leaf, eyebright is well suited for eye complaints. In the center of the lovely white flower can be found a dark spot, signifying, according to herbalists, the iris of the eye.

THE SLANTBOARD

One of the easiest and most delightful ways of getting stimulation to the upper part of the body, removing fatigue lines from the face, and bringing a flush of color to the cheeks and a sparkle to the eyes is through daily use of the slantboard, which can be simply a straight board the length and width of your body. This device will refresh the weariest person in a shorter time than is required to take a nap.

Blood flow is reversed in this head-lower-than-body position, and in consequence is forced into those very areas that are quickest to show fatigue. A headstand produces the same results, but one has to lead up to the proper headstand gradually through weeks of preparation in order to strengthen the neck muscles and learn body balance. The slantboard offers instant benefits and can be practiced at any time.

By reversing the flow of blood, the slantboard corrects sagging facial muscles and unattractive shoulder slump. It is even beneficial for varicose veins, because when you are upside down, the pressure of clogged leg veins is relieved. Fifteen minutes in the afternoon spent lying on this flat board can revitalize a fatigued body and mind and give greater zest to the remainder of the day.

What is the magic here (for no one arises from a quarter of an hour on a slantboard without realizing a return of earlier enthusiasm, coupled with a serenity you might not have known all day)?

Muscles relax when you lie in this prone, tilted position. Not the least benefit is the increased circulation to starved or under-nourished hair roots. Since this is the most difficult area of the body to stimulate, the slantboard is of great value to anyone with scalp or hair trouble. A clearer mind and complexion and a stimulated body, then, are the main benefits here.

Slantboards are available in the stores. But if you don't care to buy one, use your ironing board, folded flat. Place one end on a stable pile of books about one and one half feet high. The other end rests on the floor. Now, take a position with your head on the lower end, and stretch your body the length of the board. Relax and allow your arms to rest comfortably beside you.

This is an excellent time to use a facial or a mask, for the added blood circulation will increase its value. Use the slantboard daily for a minimum of 15 minutes. Even better are two 15-minute periods, one in midmorning and another in midafternoon.

CHAPPED HANDS

Hands must be dipped daily into moisturizing and protective creams if they are to remain attractive and comfortable. Certain foods will relieve raw, rough hands, control the effects of exposure to the elements or housework, and supply plumping and nourishing factors.

A workday cream which protects overused hands is a great investment. The sweet almond oil in the following formula offers soothing, softening, and healing qualities, while the wax holds the oil in place and, combined with it, acts as an effective covering against housework and chill winds.

Hand Cream for Winter Months

Set a glass custard cup in a pan of hot water. Drop in a 1-ounce cake of white beeswax and allow it to melt. Blend in 2 ounces of sweet almond oil. Remove from the heat and pour the contents into a glass jar. Keep this beside the sink and dip into it after any household chore. Or use it prior to going outdoors in cold weather.

CLEANSING CREAM OIL FOR FEBRUARY

This is not the month to scrub away at the face with soap and water. Whenever possible, substitute another cleansing agent in order to avoid removing protective oils from the skin. Golden nut and vegetable oils in combination create a very effective makeup remover and skin cleanser and really seem to remove more grime than any soap. And as you are cleansing away your makeup, you are adding something beneficial to your complexion when you use this oil-base cleanser.

Cleansing Cream Oil

3 tablespoons sesame seed oil
1 tablespoon sweet almond oil
1 tablespoon wheat germ oil

1 tablespoon olive oil
½ teaspoon of apple cider vinegar

Beat all ingredients together thoroughly or pour into a bottle, cap it, and shake vigorously. Blot away excess oil, and the oil is quite comfortable to keep on the face for hours. But it must eventually be removed with warm water and gently rubbed away, then the face should be splashed with cool water and dried. This oil can be used to remove makeup, to apply at night, or to wear around the house during the day.

SHAMPOO FOR DRY HAIR

A bouncy, live head of hair must be worked for in February. With weeks yet to go of cold raw weather, lack of sunshine, and additional amounts of pollution from winter soots in the air, cleansing, brightening, and pampering the hair is a February must.

Glossy hair begins with good nutrition and is maintained by the cleansing of each hair strand. But when the hair is dry, do not add insult to injury by using an indifferent or caustic shampoo. Study your hair and determine its needs.

If it is dry, then add a tablespoon of cold processed salad oil to your diet each day. It can be used on a salad, but it's better to take it directly from the spoon in order not to lose any of it. Use a shampoo that will not strip the hair of its precious oils. In fact, a soapless shampoo made from egg yolks is probably the best selection for a depleted and lifeless head of hair. And it nourishes, conditions, and brings luster to every hair strand, even as it cleanses.

Egg Yolk Shampoo for Dry Hair

Beat 2 egg yolks into 1 cup of warm—not hot—water and blend thoroughly. After brushing the hair one hundred strokes, massage a little of the mixture at a time into both hair and scalp. Do not miss any area. Set a timer, or watch a clock, and continue to massage the egg yolk into the hair and scalp for a full 5 minutes.

Place a plastic bag over your scalp and allow the rich protein mixture to soak into the dry hair shafts for another 5 minutes. Rinse the hair carefully until the water runs clear without any foam or bubble. Rinsing must be thorough for the shampoo to be effective.

OILY HAIR SHAMPOO

Use an herbal or castile shampoo and scrub both hair and scalp through two shampoos. Rinse with a final solution of one quart of warm water to which is added one tablespoon of apple cider vinegar, and towel dry. With cotton pads, apply diluted witch hazel to the hair and massage gently into the scalp. This treatment should cut down on the need for too-frequent shampoos.

HERBAL TOOTHPOWDER FOR FEBRUARY

Now when there is less fresh fruit to eat and carbohydrates seem heavy in your diet, have you looked into the mirror to check the gleam of your teeth? When strawberries, cherries, peaches, and other acidic fruits are available, you can count on their natural cleansing and brightening effects, but during February, perhaps you should increase your apple consumption and check your tooth cleanser.

There are those who feel that a toothpaste, for all its foam and flavor (plus its sometimes-objectionable ingredients) cannot really cleanse the teeth in as effective a manner as a toothpowder. In case you'd like to experiment a bit on your own and especially if you've grown doubtful of the results of using the hard-sell commercial products that are aimed at you, here is yesterday's answer to today's modern dentifrice. You can use an electric nut mill to bridge the time gap and make preparation easier.

Herbal Toothpowder

2 tablespoons powdered rosemary	1 teaspoon powdered orris root
1 teaspoon powdered myrrh	1 teaspoon powdered Peruvian bark

Grind the ingredients in an electric nut grinder and sift through a fine gauze. Store in a tightly closed wide-mouthed bottle. Shake out a sufficient quantity in your palm, wet your toothbrush, and cleanse away. The taste may not be rousing, but the results are great.

FACIAL PACK FOR DRY SKIN

Beat 1 fertilized egg yolk with 1 teaspoon of raw honey. Add ½ teaspoon of wheat germ oil and ½ teaspoon of fresh cream. Blend thoroughly and apply to a face and throat which first have been cleansed with cotton pads dipped into milk.

Gently massage the honey-egg pack onto all areas of the face and throat. When the first layer dries, add another, continuing to massage in until the face and neck have three layers of the pack.

When the layers have dried completely, remove with warm water, then cool, without using any soap. Blot dry. Repeat daily for the best effects.

FACIAL STIMULATION FOR COLOR

Wintertime weather must be countered with extra attention for the skin, or else the grayness of this time of year may match your complexion during these cheerless months. Without enough outdoor activity and sunshine to tinge a cheek with color and stimulate the body to its peak performance, skin tones can become pale and characterless. You must make your own sunshine now by using stimulating facials which help to increase the blood circulation and bring more color to the face.

Fuller's Earth is a soft, absorbent substance which will answer the purpose here. This powdery earth gives a beneficial massage to fatigued skin. Coming as it does from the earth itself, it mixes easily with liquid and can be applied in a workable paste to the face. Its greatest value seems to be in its contracting qualities that, as the powdered earth dries, create greater blood movement just beneath its covering. When an herbal tea is mixed with the paste, even greater benefits occur, according to the herb used.

Tightening of the skin takes place as the Fuller's Earth dries and hardens to a white, chalky substance. After its use, the complexion glows with color from the increased stimulation.

Fuller's Earth Pack

Mix together enough Fuller's Earth and plain yogurt to form a workable paste. To this, add 1 teaspoon of fennel tea. To prepare the fennel tea, simmer 1 tablespoon of fennel seeds in ½ cup of water for 5 minutes. Strain and use 1 teaspoon of the strong infusion for the mask. Dilute the remainder of the tea with enough mineral water to make 1 cup and use as a facial rinse to prevent wrinkles.

Spread the soft, fluid mixture across the face, avoiding the eye area entirely. Do not use any facial muscles after the pack is applied, as it will crack the mask and lessen its value. Lie down for ten to fifteen minutes as the mask dries. Rinse away with warm and then cool water. After the mask, apply a thin coating of salad oil to the skin.

To vary the earth pack, you might try mixing the earth with enough witch hazel to create a spreading consistency and proceed as above. This is better for oily and normal skins than for dry ones because of its own drying qualities.

HAIR CONDITIONING
BEFORE A SHAMPOO

It is not practical these days simply to give yourself a shampoo, for the hair is no longer a mere covering of the scalp as it once was. As an adornment and background for a woman's appearance, an incredible array of items on the market invite you to change its color and texture and burn it into curls. Today frequent repair treatments are vital to assure good hair condition. The following honey hair conditioning can do much to restore life to damaged hair and coax it back to health.

Honey Hair Conditioning

| 1 egg yolk | 1 cup raw honey |
| ½ cup cold processed olive oil | |

Beat the egg yolk into the oil and then slowly blend the oil and egg mixture into the honey.

Brush your hair thoroughly and then massage the mixture into both scalp and hair. Place a plastic bag over your hair and allow the scalp and hair to soak in this conditioner for at least 30 minutes. Shampoo your hair twice to remove the unabsorbed oil. Rinse thoroughly; add dash of apple cider vinegar or lemon juice to last rinse. Use about 1 tablespoon to 1 quart of warm water.

TO MAKE AN IPSWICH BALL

Since Cardinal Wolsey of Ipswich carried around a delicately scented pomander ball with him to offset less than agreeable odors, it is quite possible that he promoted the famous Ipswich Ball, or perfumed soap. In any event, this lively port town in England appears to be the birthplace of the traditional formula that comes in its original instructions from *The Queen's Closet Opened*, by W. M. Cook to Queen Henrietta Maria, 1655.

You can find the modern Ipswich Ball in soap departments, hanging by a rope, strand, or cord, ready to be suspended near a shower head. Retain something of the original scent and charm by making one yourself and capture something of yesterday.

Take 1 pound of fine white castile soap, shave it thin, and let it stand two or three days in a pint of rose water. Strain the water; add ½ pint of fresh water and let it stand one more day. Pour that off and add ½ pint of fresh water; let it stand another day.

Add to this ½ ounce of sweet marjoram powder, ¼ ounce of winter savory herb, ground into a powder, 2 drops of Patchouli, 2 drops of oil of cloves, ¼ teaspoon tincture of musk, and 3 teaspoons of almond meal. (Coming from an East Indian herb, Patchouli's heavy scented oil is prized in Bali, Java, and Malaya because of its ability to mask perspiration odors—a well scented Ipswich Ball may cut down on your need for additional deodorant.) Work this all together and form a ball in your hands. Allow to dry for a week before using.

APHRODISIAC FOR FEBRUARY

This is the month to mix a potent brew to return the fires of summer to a cold skin—at least, according to some herbalists. An ancient formula, this herbal body lotion is said to have brought amours aplenty to those who used it as a body wash. Let's resurrect it during this cold month of February and see what happens. To be prepared, make it during January and have it ready for February.

The recipe alone reads like a page from a sorcerer's manual. In combination, the delightful ingredients are considered strengthening, invigorating, and stimulating. Rosemary's aromatic oil has figured in concoctions for many centuries, and has its own wealth of followers around the world. Mint has been considered an aphrodisiac, and balm, or melissa, gives off a delicate lemony scent which is reminiscent of a crushed bed of cool grass on a summer's day.

Body Lotion to Inspire Passion

For this unusual and ancient preparation, use the following items.

1½ cups dried rosemary
    leaves
2 tablespoons dried mint
2 tablespoons dried balm, or
    melissa

2 tablespoons grated fresh
    lemon peel
2 tablespoons grated fresh
    orange peel
1 pint rose water mixed with
1 pint ethyl alcohol

Macerate the first five ingredients in the rose water and alcohol for a month, then filter and use. Rub sparingly on the body.

BREAKFASTS FOR FEBRUARY

Stewed dried fruit combination
Poached egg
Whole wheat toast with nut butter*
Herbal tea

Cranberry juice
Millet cereal*
Herbal tea

Natural fruit jam*
Omelet with parsley
Whole grain toast
Herbal tea

Stewed prunes
Melted cheese on whole grain bread
Herbal tea

Sliced fresh oranges
Grated apple mixed with presoaked oatmeal and ground nuts*
Herbal tea

Fresh grapefruit
Soft-boiled egg
Nut butter sandwich*
Herbal tea

Bananas and wheat germ in milk
Cornmeal chapaties and honey (recipe on p. 23)
Herbal tea

LUNCHES FOR FEBRUARY

❧

Sunburst salad of greens, fresh pineapple, bananas, and oranges
Nut butter sandwiches*
Yogurt

Celery and carrot juice cocktail
Garbanzo salad with chopped onions*
Corn muffins
Yogurt

Avocado and banana salad with homemade mayonnaise
Yogurt soup*

Beet and hard-boiled egg salad
Onion soup (recipe on p. 94)
Yogurt

Puree of string bean soup*
Black bread and cheese
Yogurt

Cream of broccoli soup*
Egg salad with rye toast
Yogurt

Vegetable soup
Sprout salad*
Yogurt

DINNERS FOR FEBRUARY

Sautéed brains
Squash with lemon and oil
Peas and onions

Baked fish
Broiled cherry tomatoes and mushrooms
Baked potato

Walnut loaf*
Braised cabbage
Fresh beets with grated orange rind

Sautéed liver dipped in wheat germ
Chopped fresh cherry tomatoes and parsley
Brown rice with oil and lemon

Stuffed eggplant*
String beans, lima, and celery combination

Ground beef and beef heart patties
Parsnips
Turnip greens

Baked eggs with mushrooms*
Cauliflower
Zucchini squash

RECIPES FOR FEBRUARY

Nut Butter

1 cup nutmeats   honey
oil

Grind nuts until they are fine and mealy. Blend in enough nut or vegetable oil to make a paste; add honey to sweeten.

Variation: Put ½ cup dried apricots, raisins, and water-softened prunes through grinder and blend with nut butter.

Millet Cereal

1 cup milk   ½ teaspoon salt
1 cup water   2 tablespoons honey
½ cup hulled millet

Place water and milk in upper part of double boiler and bring to a boil. Slowly stir in millet and salt and simmer for 5 minutes over direct heat. Place over lower part of double boiler, cover, and steam for 30 minutes. Add honey and serve with milk.

Natural Fruit Jam

½ pound dried pears 1 cup raisins
½ pound dried apricots honey
½ pound dried, pitted prunes

Rinse fruit and soak overnight with water to cover. Cook the prunes in the soaking water and put all fruit through the grinder on a fine blade. Stir in enough honey to bind and sweeten.

Grated Apple, Oatmeal, and Nuts

1 cup rolled oats juice of one orange
1 grated apple, with skin honey to taste
¼ cup chopped nutmeats ½ cup nut, seed, or soy milk

Mix ingredients and allow to stand overnight, covered, to soften.

Garbanzo Salad

1 cup cooked garbanzos ½ cup chopped fresh tomatoes
¼ cup chopped onions ¼ cup minced parsley
¼ cup minced green pepper 1 tablespoon salad oil

Mix ingredients and allow to blend for 3 hours or more.

Yogurt Soup

2 cucumbers, chopped dill
2 cups yogurt garlic
2 tablespoons lemon juice

Place cucumbers, yogurt, and lemon juice in blender; add dill and garlic to season. Blend to a smooth consistency and serve cold.

Puree of String Bean Soup

1 cup quickly cooked string
    beans
1 cup chicken broth

½ cup milk
seasoning

Place all ingredients together in blender and reduce to a soupy consistency. Add more milk if a thinner soup is desired. Heat just below a simmer and serve.

Cream of Broccoli Soup

Cook broccoli with chopped onion just until tender and add with milk to the blender. Liquefy and sprinkle with grated Swiss cheese.

Sprout Salad

1 cup mung sprouts
1 chopped apple

1 cup shredded romaine or
    Chinese cabbage
¼ cup sunflower meal

Season ingredients with a vegetable salt and sprinkle with oil and lemon juice.

Walnut Loaf

1 cup chopped walnuts
1 cup dried whole wheat
    crumbs
1 cup minced celery
½ cup chopped green pepper

½ cup chopped onion
2 tablespoons vegetable oil
1 beaten egg
1 cup tomato juice
sea salt

Mix ingredients together and bake in oiled loaf pan for 1 hour at 375 degrees.

Stuffed Eggplant

1 eggplant
1 cup cooked chicken
½ cup wheat germ
1 cup chopped tomatoes
¼ cup chopped onion

¼ cup minced parsley
¼ cup vegetable oil
1 teaspoon fresh or dried sage
1 beaten egg
sea salt

Cut eggplant in half and steam just until interior is soft to the touch. Scoop out the inner section and mix with other ingredients. Return to the shell and bake for 45 minutes at 375 degrees.

Baked Eggs with Mushrooms

1 dozen mushrooms
3 tablespoons vegetable oil
lemon juice
sea salt
1 cup chicken stock

arrowroot
6 eggs
½ cup whole wheat bread-
crumbs
parsley

Sauté mushrooms in oil, add lemon juice and salt, and cook covered for 5 minutes. Thicken stock with arrowroot and add to mushrooms, cook an additional 5 minutes. Remove from heat and blend in beaten eggs. Pour into a buttered baking dish and cover with crumbs and parsley. Bake in a hot oven until the eggs are set, about 5 minutes. Serve immediately.

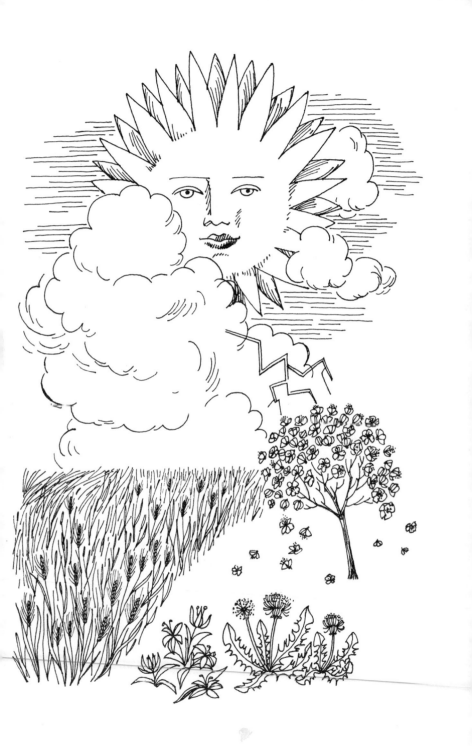

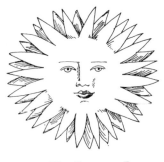

March

Ah, March! We know thou art
Kind hearted, spite of ugly looks and
threats
And, out of sight, art nursing April's
violets!

Helen Hunt: "March"

In point of origin, this month's name comes from Mars. The Saxons had a word for it that wasn't particularly kind—Rough-Month, because of its boisterous winds. The French calendar repeated the thought in Windy Month.

And what needs doing now? Well, what has winter done to your hands? Are they soft and beautiful and competent-looking, or only competent-looking? Lather them with honey and water. Massage rich honey and sweet almond oil into them. Dip them into softening bran water and extravagantly bathe your entire body in a whole tub of this old-fashioned magic. Remove the pale of January and February by stimulating the skin with a freshening almond meal cleanser. Gather dandelion for food and cosmetic.

Cleanse the blood and remove sallow skin tones. Acknowledge the coming rebirth of the earth by looking under leaf and bush until you spot the first crocus and quivering hyacinth. And plan to join this resurgence of life by giving special attention to your own spring self.

PROTEIN SKIN FOOD
AND WRINKLE REDUCER

With a glance backward, try whipping up an old-fashioned rejuvenating brew of pure protein which, while it is on your skin, returns the appearance of youth to the face. Lines and wrinkles disappear under the application of this double-rich skin food. When the mask dries, years seem to drop from your appearance. Unfortunately, this is only temporary, for it is not a comfortable covering to wear for longer than it needs to dry. Even so, once rinsed away many benefits remain. The skin has been nourished and stimulated by the tautening action of the mixture and is more resilient with a lessening of line depth. By applying this paste, you have furnished a potent food to starved skin, and the results are indeed rewarding. And the incredibly active drying process stimulates your face by bringing fresh blood supplies which help both to cleanse and nourish.

Mix 2 teaspoons of soy protein powder with 1 teaspoon of egg yolk and 1 tablespoon of water. Beat together until thoroughly blended and spread evenly in a thin layer over the face and throat. Leave on to dry, around 30 minutes. If possible, do not speak or smile or use any facial muscles while the mask is on. Rinse away with warm water, then dash cool water across the face. Blot dry and apply a thin coating of oil if your skin feels dry.

EXERCISES FOR REVITALIZING

The streamlined approach to beauty must include daily exercise. Without it the body will rebel, will not be lithe and sleek, and will manifest signs of age more swiftly than seems possible. The beautiful girl of twenty will appear, at age twenty-five without exercise, a bit too voluptuous and more mature than she wishes. At thirty, if she still hasn't formulated a daily exercise routine, the softness of body form will probably have assumed unflattering proportions, and she will be hiding behind uncomfortable girdles and A-line dresses.

As the years go on and this underexercised woman continues to throw away her youth, bodily ills may accompany her sedentary ways. Certainly, if she goes through her entire life without the beneficial results of planned body movements, she has literally squandered her beauty and a great deal of increased joy she could have known from a splendidly functioning body.

Exercises improve both mind and body. An uncomfortable body quickly produces a harried, irritable mind. And the results of the latter can etch permanent frown lines and sagging flesh folds into the skin. The perpetual frowner, the squinter, and the generally disquieted person is especially susceptible to early aging signs.

If you have avoided an exercise program because you hate vigorous physical activity, there are exercises you can perform with no more physical exertion than walking across a room. Not everyone is geared to athletics. And because of this, many people develop poorly functioning bodies in the mistaken belief that exercise must be a series of frenzied body movements in order to be effective.

Not so. Yoga and exercises based on this discipline offer a gentle body flexing stimulation which can tone the weariest limbs and restore lines of beauty lost to easy living and indifference.

Easy exercising will condition and revitalize the aging and uncomfortable person and bring the color of life to characterless skin which has been starved by a sluggish bloodstream. Stiffness, associated with aging, can happen even to young people. Yet the easy exercising in this book can actually reverse those signs if practiced on a daily basis. Good circulation, which speaks of good health, can be achieved by simple and easy exercises.

In fact, a woman practicing her exercises daily, without fail, will be able to flip back the calendar pages in her personal appearance long before the end of the year if she is dedicated enough to work for a youthful body.

She can become a beautiful person with no additional asset, other than the way she controls her body. When such a woman enters or leaves a room, people are aware of her presence even if she has done no more than pass through. This woman values her body. It will not embarrass her or otherwise irritate or annoy her.

Head high and stately, no matter what her size, the well-exercised body will be carried easily in movement and will not sidle, lope, stumble, or present itself unattractively. There is a pride of movement in a beautifully exercised woman. She owns herself, but in a relaxed and casual manner which frees her to acknowledge and join the world, completely putting herself from mind.

CARE OF THE HANDS

Rubber gloves are one of the greatest aids in beauty care. Hands can deal with all the drudgery of work necessary, and if gloves are worn, the hands will come away as shapely and smooth as if they hadn't a sign of wear on them.

Certainly, in this day of detergents it is vital to keep the hands out of strong cleansing solutions. Doctors have found among their patients women whose hands and nails are so badly damaged by the frequent use of modern cleansers that nail loss and serious abrasion of skin tissue develop. These conditions usually clear up when the hands are kept out of the harsh solutions.

But gloves permit the use of these caustic products without harm to the skin. While it is difficult for some women to learn to work in rubber gloves, it will be a practice well learned if you want to retain attractive hands and nails.

Hands are very revealing of age. All too soon the skin will seem to shrink and dry unless pampered and nourished with external applications of rich, moisture-bearing creams and oils. One might think hand care posed a greater problem in earlier days than now, but though housework might have been harder and more demanding, there were no harmful sprays and detergents on the market then. Even so, early instructions for good hand care usually advised herbal, fruit, and vegetable lotions and waxes containing everything from lanolin to oatmeal.

While there are coverups for the face and its occasional blemishes, there is very little you can do to conceal damaged hands. Too late in the day you usually remember the hands, and then a quick squirt of useless lotion, probably laced with glycerin, is rubbed hastily into the skin.

Hand care should and must begin in the kitchen, for it is here that most of the crimes against attractive hands are committed. Extremes of water temperature drain out the scant oil supplies and chill and contract the skin, and in addition the hands are seldom dried thoroughly enough after immersion in water.

One English beautician, when teaching hand care, stresses the need to dry the hands thoroughly after washing them. And she suggests that few people really dry their hands to the degree necessary to prevent redness, chapping, and drying of the outer skin. It is her belief that many unattractive and raw-looking hand conditions could be avoided by this one good practice.

According to another beautician, the best effects of applying hand cream can be achieved only if the cream is worked into the hands while they are under very warm water. Lotions would not be useful in this method. But a waxy, heat-expanding, and penetrating cream should work very well. Honey and oil hand cream would be ideal for this. And as a matter of fact, this cream requires the immersion in hot water to be effective by allowing the wax to spread and cover and soothe.

Daily care is simple enough, if the practice is made easy by keeping a supply of the protective cream necessary for good hand treatment around. Many of the items that will turn work-roughened hands into softer-skinned ones are on your kitchen shelves right now. There are others which you should have if you are really serious about the care of your body. And few of the items will cost more than pennies a recipe.

Bran has been used for centuries as a skin softener. In earlier days, women not only used bran water as a delightful hand lotion, but applied it to the face and drank a daily broth made from it to clear the blood.

SOFT BRAN WATER FOR THE HANDS

Boil 1 cup of bran for 5 minutes in enough water to make a thin gruel. Strain the mixture into a container and keep some of it beside the washbasin. Refrigerate the remainder. Each time you wash your hands, pour some of this liquid into a glass, mix with a bit of water, and use it as a rinse for the hands, massaging it thoroughly into the skin before blotting the hands dry.

Honey is also generous with qualities for the overworked and undercared-for hands. Smoothing, healing, and softening, this golden amber liquid can restore hands that have become dried into a caricature of themselves.

Sweet almond oil has been used for centuries by women around the world and is especially helpful when mixed with egg yolk and honey to form a thick cream which nourishes the skin.

The wealth of rich nutrients in almond oil was made possible by a whim that turned into an industry. A Portuguese king once married a beautiful Scandinavian princess and brought her to sunny Portugal to live. The new queen was so homesick for her lost land of snow that she wept by the hour. The saddened king ordered almond trees to be planted as far as the eye could see, hoping the beauty of the trees in blossom would assuage his lonely queen.

And, of course, one morning the queen looked out of her window to find the entire countryside covered with white. It was the almond trees in bloom, and the queen became peaceful and lived happily ever after. Or at least, in the springtime, when the almond blossoms paved her sweeping grounds.

But with all those trees, and consequent crops of almonds, the oil from the sweet nuts was put to use, and some clever woman discovered if she wore the oil as well as cooked with it, she increased her beauty tenfold.

Honey and Oil Cream

½ ounce white wax
½ ounce spermaceti, available from a botanical supply house

8 ounces honey
1 ounce sweet almond oil
perfumed oil or perfume

Place the wax and spermaceti in a container over hot water. Allow them to dissolve, and then beat in the honey and almond oil. When everything is mixed well, remove from the heat and allow to cool somewhat before adding the perfume and pouring into a glass jar.

Use this exquisite concoction instead of soap. Run very warm water into the wash basin, dip into the honey and oil cream and massage the cream into the hands while they are under water. While hands are still warm, blot them dry.

BRAN BATH FOR MARCH

The stripping winds of March can be just as severe as the colder winter months. And just as damaging to your body's skin. If you have lavished care on your body and protected it against dry heated rooms, and their opposite in stinging cold weather by adding natural oils and foods containing these oils to both bath and diet, then continue this good care in the form of a bran bath which will add its own oils and vegetable hormones to protect the skin covering.

A rich addition to the bath, bran can be used in a variety of ways. This outer coating of the wheat kernel has been used as a face wash for centuries by women seeking softer skin. With its concentrated amounts of vitamin B and rich minerals, bran makes a bath solution that can combat rough texture and the scaliness of abused and dry skin if used frequently.

Tie 1 cup of bran in a muslin or gauze bag and swish it around in the water. Or, place 2 cups of the bran in 2 quarts of cold water. Bring it to a slow simmer and hold it at that temperature for 5 minutes. Strain and mash in order to extract all moisture. Pour this into a tub half filled with water. Fill a drawstring bag or the end of a nylon stocking with the leftover mash and use it to scour the body and give a fine luster to the skin.

FACIAL CLEANSER FOR MARCH

New skin is just as eager to show itself as the first violets or the crisp little dandelion leaves in the springtime. But it is seldom permitted to come forth, padded and covered as it is by impacted powder bases, residue cold creams, and blushers, tints, and gels. Though the skin tissue does indeed renew itself, it usually must first be stripped of the outer debris that accumulates from hasty and insufficient cleansing.

The freshness of new facial skin is enormously rewarding. Weariness, fatigue, and even age seem to peel off with the lifting of the dead scarf skin that creates so many cosmetic problems.

You can greet the budding spring season with a new skin by using a sweet almond meal cleanser, and produce a radiantly clean face for this freshening month.

Sweet Almond Meal Cleanser

Blanch a quarter cup of almonds. Place in a nut grinder or blender and reduce to a fine powder. Be sure the nuts are completely dry before attempting to grind them. Mix the almond meal with one teaspoon of sweet almond oil and enough milk to make a paste. Pat onto a freshly scrubbed and moist face and allow to dry. With a damp washcloth, rub gently in upward motions until the cleanser is removed. Rinse the face well in warm and then cool water. Pat on a thin film of oil if the skin is dry.

STIMULATING YEAST MASK

A beauty food which can restore rosiness to cheeks, bring a flush of life, and give a positive glow to ailing skin can be put together as a mask and used weekly for those who face the month of March with a leftover winter look.

Brewer's yeast is a must in the diet and beauty plan of any woman who knows the requirements of health. A magnificent source of the B vitamins, vital to skin beauty, brewer's yeast also contains amino acids and minerals. A high protein product, this miracle food can help rid you of pallor and grayness of skin that result from poor circulation. For the best results, it should be taken internally at the same time it is applied as a face mask.

Start by stirring 1 teaspoon of yeast into a glass of tomato juice three times a day and drinking it. Over a period of time, work up to 3 level tablespoons of the yeast a day. Apply the following mask twice a week for the best results.

Yeast Mask

1 tablespoon brewer's yeast   3 tablespoons milk
   in powder form

Mix together into a paste and apply to a clean face and neck. Allow the mixture to dry on the skin 15 to 30 minutes, as required. Loosen by steaming slightly with a washcloth dipped into warm water.

Gently rub at the face and neck to remove all traces of the mask. If your skin is dry, apply a thin film of salad oil and blot away any excess. Do not speak or use the facial muscles in any way until the mask has fully dried, for the yeast mask not only nourishes and stimulates the skin, but smooths out—if only temporarily—little lines and wrinkles.

When used on the throat area, always rub in a cream or oil as this is a particularly dry part of the body, as is the area around the eyes. While the yeast mask stimulates this area, you must at the same time replace the scant oil supply absorbed by it.

DANDELION WASH FOR MARCH

Who says the dandelion should not take equal honors with the crocus and snowdrop? And who, knowing the incredible goodness and beauty of the dandelion, can really dislike its generous appearance on each and every lawn, field, and byway? Held in low esteem in the gardener's manual, this plant is a veritable treasure in the beauty book. The graceful, saw-toothed leaves of the dandelion should occupy a throne in the kingdom of beauty preparations.

Why this accolade for one of nature's seemingly cruel jokes on the enthusiastic lawnkeeper? For one, it is a blood cleanser with few if any equals. When the tiny serrated leaves appear early in March, every woman who is concerned with her own beauty and her family's health should be out with pan and knife, cutting the crisp emerald leaves to mix with other greens in a spring salad. As a tonic, the dandelion has been advocated by herbalists for centuries. As it grows and matures, the plant becomes too bitter to be eaten. March is the time to gather the larger leaves and use them as a facial wash.

A good source of vitamin A, the dandelion also has vitamin B, some C, G, iron, potassium, magnesium, silicon, and calcium— beauty vitamins and minerals all. Invaluable as a face wash, the dandelion will help remove sallowness and strengthen the facial tissues at the same time with its cleansing and purifying effects.

DANDELION FACIAL PACK

Pick a cupful of young tender dandelion leaves and mince them. Place in 1½ cups cold water and slowly bring to a boil. Simmer for 10 minutes, covered; then allow the liquid to cool to lukewarm. Apply the softened herbal mixture to a double piece of gauze and place the square on your face when you lie down, preferably on a slantboard, for 15 to 20 minutes. Rinse away with warm, then cool, water and blot dry.

This facial pack should be used at least three times a week for the entire month. Prepare the pack from fresh leaves each time. Your lawn will be smoother, and so will your skin. This preparation is also noted for removing lines from the face.

For those who simply won't take the time to lie down under the dandelion pack, prepare a wash for your face from the same brew. Simply mash and strain the stewed dandelion leaves through a strainer and apply the liquid to the skin several times a day, not venturing outdoors until the liquid dries on the skin.

COCONUT CREAM FOR THE HAIR

Here is an unusual but effective shampoo if you have problem hair and nothing has ever given it a nice gloss. The preparation is not as easy to use as opening a plastic bottle and pouring a liquid over the hair. But then, you haven't been able to get such great results from that, so perhaps this is what you have been looking for. This formula is for those who care to do their very best by their hair.

An old and cherished formula, it comes from a lovely Chinese woman who lives in Sumatra and who is modern enough to swing with the times and send several sons and daughters out into the world beautifully equipped with an education she guided. She herself, however, clings to her known customs on personal care, and this is one of the beauty secrets she has practiced all her life, as did her mother and grandmother before her.

She shares this formula for hair beauty with you, and hopes you have the patience to prepare it, in order to see its rich rewards.

Coconut Shampoo

Drain coconut water from the shell and remove the shell itself by heating in an oven at 100 degrees until the shell cracks and can be slipped off. Place coconut in blender in small pieces, a few at a time, and reduce to a pulp. Strain the pulp through gauze to obtain the thick coconut cream.

Take a lemon that has been slightly heated or left at room temperature for some hours, and rub it against a metal-edged glass or container in order to release the oil in the peel. Mix this oil with the coconut cream squeezed from the pulp. Rub this combination into the hair and scalp and leave on for 15 minutes. Wash out with an herbal shampoo and use lemon juice or a dollop of apple cider vinegar in the last rinse.

This charming lady says that in her homeland hair was dried by placing a bamboo pole over a chair and beating the hair over the bamboo; this was supposed to both strengthen and dry it. I suggest sitting in the sun or towel drying, instead.

ABDOMINAL EXERCISES

March is not too early to start thinking about a summertime figure. In fact, there will just be time now, with daily exercises, to pare the body down, to firm uncertain flesh, and to create a beautiful figure which can fit into a bathing suit without bulging out of every opening.

Each year we all make resolutions to prepare our bodies for

summertime comfort, but because it seems like such a project, the resolutions are seldom carried out. But if March is here, can June be far behind? It is now or never, if you really want a summer body which can give you comfort and pride.

What areas bulge in a bathing suit? Thighs, abdomen, shoulders, arms. Let's begin with the abdomen, for you cannot try a bathing suit until this is firmed to the flatness that will permit you to drop down a size or two if you are heavy in this area.

The bulging flesh of the stomach region is due in part to weakened muscles in the abdominal wall. This softened flesh presents a most unattractive appearance, and can ruin the lines of an otherwise perfect body. Muscles alone can hold this fleshy region in position if they are in good condition. If you do not commit yourself to a regular plan of exercise, the slight pot will increase in time to a mountainous bulge.

Exercise will elasticize the soft abdominal region and tone the inner organs that have grown flaccid. In time, you can develop a muscular belt which will give you not only a beautiful body profile, but also a buoyancy of feeling because everything is in its right place.

Before you begin exercising, study your problem areas. Stand nude before a full-length mirror and honestly take stock. Turn sideways, standing comfortably in your usual position, and regard your body profile.

Mentally record those areas most in need of redemption. Usually, the abdomen is the greatest offender. But remember, it is only what you have made it. You started out with a flat, attractive stomach. Lean and lovely. What happened? Too little exercise and too many cream puffs or other pastries? The problem can be corrected if you are brave enough and regard your body as the living temple it really is.

Begin your exercises casually. If you start with a full-steam-ahead attitude, it may dwindle because it is hard to sustain excessive enthusiasm.

The abdominal roll is really a pleasant, uncomplicated, and immensely effective body movement. Because the abdomen is a difficult area to reach in exercising, you must use involuntary muscles to shape and tone the abdominal wall. The stomach roll uses these muscles to pull in, roll over, under, and sideways in this center region.

Results can be astounding. Elimination can become easier and more punctual, flabby skin tightens, and comfortable and correct posture is possible.

Abdominal Roll

Stand upright with your knees slightly bent and your legs apart. Visualize your stomach as a ball and draw in your breath, pulling the stomach in with this action toward the spine. Hold it there a moment, and then lift the imaginary ball that is the stomach upward to its highest point before rolling it over and down.

Visualize the ball making a complete turn within the entire area that is your abdomen. Start slowly with this exercise, but after the first week repeat it several times during the day.

More difficult, but of additional value, is the contracting of muscles to cause the "ball" that is your stomach to go from left to right in a sideways circle. Reverse in a right to left pattern.

Reducing the Abdomen

Lie flat on the floor, face down. Place your palms on the floor just below shoulder level with your elbows pointed slightly outward. Take a deep breath and very slowly push upward on the palms to lift your head, shoulders, and abdomen as far back as you comfortably can. Exhale and slowly lower yourself to the floor again. The palms should not move, but remain in the same position, both going up and coming down. The backward pull of this exercise helps tone the oversized abdomen and stimulates the internal organs and muscles.

Another abdominal exercise uses a pulling method to gain good muscle tone. Lie flat on the floor on your back with your arms by your sides. Bend your right knee and lift your leg ceilingward until your toes are pointing directly overhead. Bend your knee and slowly drop your foot to the floor directly in front of you. Slide the foot along the floor until your leg is once more flat. Repeat with the left leg.

APHRODISIAC FOR MARCH

Who would believe that a pinhead's worth of silicon in the body could make the difference between a great lover and a nonfunctioning one? If great lovers are made, not born, then without doubt prosaic things like cabbage, greens, and strawberries, among other healthy foods, figure in the diet in a very important way.

And figs. Desert nomads wouldn't be caught without their saddlebags filled with this delicious and sustaining food. And within this nectared fruit is silicon, a trace mineral which prevents impotence.

How about a dessert of figs mixed with cream, nuts, and rice to end a meal and begin a pleasant evening?

Celestial Figs

½ cup chopped dried figs
½ cup chopped toasted almonds

1 cup crushed pineapple
1 cup chilled cooked rice
1 cup whipped cream

Mix the first four ingredients together and fold in the cream.

BREAKFASTS FOR MARCH

Stewed apples
Millet cereal (recipe on p. 45)
Herbal tea

Mushroom omelet
Whole grain bread
Broiled tomatoes
Herbal tea

Grape juice
Soya rice waffles*
Fruit sauce
Herbal tea

Orange slices
Brown rice and raisins
Herbal tea

Sliced bananas in orange juice
Muesli and currants
Herbal tea

Cranberry juice
Corn cakes with wheat germ (recipe on p. 213)
Natural fruit jam (recipe on p. 46)
Herbal tea

Stewed dried pears
Poached eggs on oatcakes*
Herbal tea

LUNCHES FOR MARCH

❧❦❧

Cottage cheese with grated vegetables
Nut butter sandwiches (recipe on p. 45)
Yogurt

Walnut, apple, banana, and avocado salad
Peanut butter and rye crackers
Yogurt

Black bean soup
Watercress, cauliflower, almond, and green pepper salad
Yogurt

Cream of broccoli soup (recipe on p. 47)
Cheese strips, tomato wedges, zucchini slices
Yogurt

Lentil soup
Cabbage, radish, and green pepper salad
Yogurt

Marigold and chive rice
Dandelion salad*
Yogurt

Barley soup
Sprout, dandelion, and apple salad*
Yogurt

DINNERS FOR MARCH

Squash griddle cakes*
Baked fish
Raw spinach salad

Sautéed liver dipped in wheat germ
Steamed shredded beets and carrots
Baked potato

Nut loaf (recipe on p. 47)
Broccoli
Parsnips

Soybean casserole
Broiled tomatoes
String beans

Broiled kidneys
Peas
Eggplant and tomatoes

Cheese soufflé
Potatoes in skins
Dandelion greens

Stuffed peppers*
Turnips
Brown rice cooked in bouillon

RECIPES FOR MARCH

Soya Rice Waffles

1 egg, separated and beaten separately	⅔ cup brown rice flour
2 tablespoons honey	⅓ cup soya flour
2 tablespoons vegetable oil	1 tablespoon baking powder
¾ cup milk	½ tablespoon sea salt

Beat egg yolk and honey into oil and milk and blend into sifted dry ingredients. Fold in stiffly beaten egg white and bake in waffle iron.

Oatcakes

2 cups rolled oats	¼ cup vegetable oil
1 tablespoon honey	½ cup water

Grind the oats through food grinder. (Do not reduce to powder by using the blender; a rough textured dough is required here.) Beat honey, oil, and water together and knead into oatmeal. Place on a floured board and roll out. Cut large biscuits and place on an oiled cookie sheet. Bake at 350 degrees for 15 to 20 minutes, until golden brown.

Dandelion Salad

1 cup young dandelion
    leaves   sea salt
1 cup fresh spinach leaves   salad oil
¼ cup chopped green onions   lemon juice

Tear the greens into bite-sized pieces, add the onions and salt, and sprinkle with oil and lemon juice.

Sprout, Dandelion, and Apple Salad

Mix together equal quantities of mung, lentil, wheat, or other sprouts with dandelion, chopped apple, and sunflower meal. Use lemon juice or apple cider vinegar and oil dressing.

Squash Griddle Cakes

potato flour   2 teaspoons baking powder
1 cup finely grated squash   1 tablespoon honey
½ cup milk   1 beaten egg
1 tablespoon oil   sea salt to taste

Beat potato flour into the squash and add milk to form a medium thick mixture. Add the other ingredients and additional potato flour if the mixture is too thin. Bake on a hot griddle.

Stuffed Peppers

1 cup diced chicken, cooked
½ cup chopped celery
½ cup cooked brown rice
2 tablespoons salad oil

½ cup tomato juice
sea salt
4 peppers, parboiled

Mix first six ingredients together and pile into peppers. Bake in oiled pan at 350 degrees for 30 minutes. If necessary, add additional tomato juice to prevent drying.

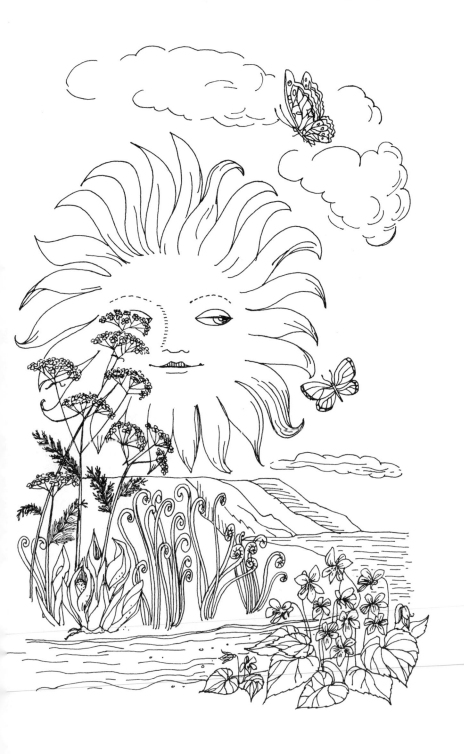

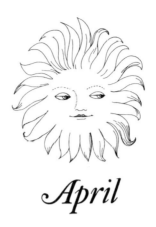

April

Come, loveliest season of the year,
And every quickened pulse shall beat,
Your footsteps in the grass to hear,
And feel your kisses soft and sweet.

Phoebe Cary: "Spring After the War"

April is universally recognized as the first month, the time of new growth and the rebirth of all living things. Called the Time of Budding in the French calendar, April makes everyone fall gladly into step with its glistening freshness. It is a world which offers so much and wants only recognition of its beauty.

Gather the first violets of the season for food and beauty. Make lotions, salads, and mouthwashes from them, and feel as fresh and delicate as the dewy blossoms themselves. Renew your body's skin by using Cleopatra's oil-scraping technique. This gentle rubbing away of surface debris after a lavish oil application can bring you the sleek body skin for which the Nile Queen was noted.

Pick a basket of chamomile to brighten your winter-dulled hair. Renew your lease on life by learning to flex your entire body. Then join the lovely promenade of spring that will carry you happily through this month and the ones to follow.

74

The first green things are up. Swamp cabbage pushes forth tentative stalks which will shortly become sturdy leaves spreading their aprons over brackish lowlands. The fiddle-neck fern spears a leftover leaf as it insistently rises from its sleeping bed. Day by day, the tightly furled frond will loosen and unfold, much as a caterpillar metamorphoses into a butterfly.

But while the butterfly takes to the air, delicately alighting now and then on stalk and vine, the fiddle-neck fern waits patiently to serve as stationary beauty aid or food, for those knowledgeable about plant life go with basket in hand and sever the tender buds before they unfold. This delicious plant tastes like asparagus, which, more deeply sleeping, waits a bit longer to sprout. So lightly steam spring's first offerings and feel the renewal of life in their fresh spring taste.

In earlier times, we were really two people—a winter person and a summer person. Deprived of green and growing food during the long, cold winter months, the winter person lived mostly on such staples as dried beans, squashes, corn, and herbs. Then came spring and he went rushing forth into the green world, snatching up all that was edible to satiate old hungers and renew his life's blood from the freshness of the growing plants.

In contrast, our food supplies change little from season to season. However, most fresh foods are trucked in from great distances and have lost much of their food value in transit. Many times we receive only a minimum of vitamins and other nutrients from tomatoes, corn, and the like because of the marketing of unripe crops and the long delay in transporting them across the country. So we should still seek out local produce and edible wild plants, and reinstate the custom of feasting on leaf and bud to supplement the mostly deficient modern diet.

WILD HERB SKIN RESTORER

April brings quickened growth to the land and there are those who say the weed must rule because these sturdier plants seem to burst forth first. Before the primrose and daisy and long before the rose and lily, the dandelion, nettle, and comfrey leaves appear. Are they stronger? Certainly they aren't considered the beauties that their delicately scented sister plants are. But much beauty lies in the strength of so-called weeds; as a wise observer once noted, "Weeds are herbs that haven't been recognized yet."

And it is the sturdy, mineral-rich wild plants—weeds, if you will—that can restore life to an ailing April skin and remove an aging gray skin tone, replacing it with a bloom. Gather a double handful each of wild strawberry leaves, with their tonic qualities, stinging nettle (be sure you are wearing gloves, for the raw leaves will sting and raise blisters if touched directly before either cooking or drying), and dandelion leaves. Wash them all and chop finely before placing in ½ cup of water and stewing gently for 10 minutes.

Place the warm mixture in a piece of gauze (double it to prevent dripping). Lie down and when prone, carefully mold the moistened herbs around your face, avoiding the eye area. Remove the herb pack after 20 minutes and rinse the face. Gently rub dry with upward circular motions. Pat on a thin covering of vegetable or nut oil and blot dry.

For those who do not have a patch of wild growth conveniently near, substitute from the herbalist's shop or botanical supply house cinquefoil, parsley, and lime flowers for the wild herbs listed. Use in the same manner to the same end.

REBUILDING THE HAIR

Probably no area of the body causes more despair than the scalp and its supposed crowning glory. When the face gradually ages, showing thread lines of wear, or blemishes and blotches, we can try to cover up, buy a new lipstick, or shrug and make the best of things.

But not so with the hair. By far the majority of letters sent to a beauty editor ask, "What shall I do about my hair?" Problems range from brittle, difficult-to-manage hair to actual balding in both women and men. Some people resign themselves to the fact that they have less than lovely hair, but this is the wrong attitude. Most hair problems can be improved or completely eliminated. And most of the improvements begin with better nutrition. There are several factors relating to good hair growth. A change in diet can bring lustrous growth to lank, indifferent strands. It can also change oily, matted hair to a halo of shining, normal hair which has the oil correctly distributed by correctly functioning glands.

It is the glands that can play mischief with the scalp and hair. If your hair is in bad condition, it is just another indication of a malfunctioning body. Seldom is the hair alone in trouble. Within or without the body there is usually another or other areas which need rehabilitation, for hair is created by the same process as all other body cells.

Thus the composition of hair has its source in an area other than the follicles that hold it. Everything you eat eventually shows its traces in the hair strand. Even medication can be found on the scalp; aspirin shows up as residue on the scalp itself within hours of your taking it.

The body was created as an exquisitely functioning mechanism, and it assumes that everything that goes into it is meant for digestion and the promotion of cellular growth or repair. There is no method by which the body can separate harmful foods from good, and shunt the undesired side effects to an area where they won't be noticed.

Bodily processes break down nourishing food into elements needed for regeneration and send them to all areas of the body. But if harmful items enter the body, the process is the same. (The body is geared for a specific work rather than casual selectivity.) Alcohol, coffee, sweets, white flour products—all leave devastating effects on the hair and the rest of the body.

It is up to the individual to make her selection of food, knowing this will, to a major degree, determine the condition not only of her body, but of her mental comfort and performance, too. Hair growth and maintenance are just as dependent on nutrition as are the skin, the organs, and the bones.

Another important factor in good hair growth is circulation. No matter how intense your interest and practice of good nutrition, if your blood vessels are so constricted they cannot carry the rich nutrients to the hair base, then your hair will continue to starve in the midst of plenty.

Food containing ample B vitamins can help improve blood circulation. This is where liver and brewer's yeast and granulated soya come in. These three foods included in an otherwise nutritionally rich diet can help correct the problem. There are other B vitamin sources, and all these foods offer benefits in addition to good hair health. Sunflower seeds eaten daily are a veritable gold mine of improved physical functions. Lecithin from soya granules, wheat germ, and egg yolk can be added to the daily diet and truly considered beauty foods contributing mightily to hair health.

A nervous disposition can result in a scanty growth of hair and can reduce a luxuriant head of hair to wispy straw. Yoga exercises practiced daily offer relief even to the person whose nerves are so bad she has long since forgotten about her hair and is merely holding on to her sanity.

The relaxing movements of this discipline bring not only

physical ease, but mental serenity, too. Your body cannot function at its best when you are agitated, and vice versa. Bodily ills and discomforts destroy composure and this in turn more deeply affects the mind. Or perhaps you have a troublesome and seemingly unsolvable problem. In time tension and inner turmoil will reflect itself in poor hair growth, whether in the form of balding spots or actual overall loss of hair.

In order to avoid this condition, learn yoga and make it a part of your daily life. While exercise alone will not magically make problems disappear, it will create a calmer, more rational, and tranquil attitude which will permit you to cope with whatever problems arise in your life.

This ancient discipline has never lost value or favor with those who recognize their body's need for moderate but daily exercise. There is no exhaustion in the practice of yoga movements. On the contrary, one is rejuvenated, exhilarated, refreshed, and calmed all at the same time. In many instances, the body and mind are healed with the continued practice of yoga.

The exercises included in each chapter of this book are variations on yogic postures and exercises, and, as such, in line with yogic beliefs, are easy to perform and rewarding in their practice.

SPRING VIOLETS
FOR EATING AND WEARING

April is the month of violets. Lovely pale or purple blossoms lift slanted buds on fragile stems and the heart-shaped leaf is the stage above which they tremble.

Violet leaves and flowers eaten in a salad or taken as a tea are supposed to soothe nerves and lessen headaches. Certainly the prettiness of the plant can bring only pleasure, and if these other attributes exist, one is the recipient of beauty plus comfort.

Gather both flowers and leaves and mix them with lettuce for a superior salad. Use only the darker violet for both its delicate scent and food and cosmetic value. Violet leaves are heavily endowed with vitamin C, and several leaves in a salad each day will assure you of a springtime source of this beauty vitamin.

Violet Salad

Crisp a bowl of freshly washed violet leaves and flowers. Add to spring lettuce and toss in separated orange slices and almonds. Use a light dressing made with lemon juice and vegetable or nut oil.

The emollient quality of both flower and leaf makes the violet invaluable for the skin. If the face is bathed in violet water daily, the softening effect can be felt within a matter of two weeks or less.

Violet Water Skin Softener

Mince 1 tablespoon of violet flowers and leaves finely and place in 1 cup of cold water. Bring to a simmer for 2 minutes, remove from the heat, and steep with a lid on until the water is just warm to the touch. Bathe the face in this liquid three or four times a day.

Another springtime delicacy is a fragrant mouthwash made with fresh violets. A great many of the flowers are required for this preparation, so take a basket, go for a long walk in the woods and meadows, along solitary pathways, and fill your basket, all the time looking forward to having breath that truly speaks of violets and spring.

Honey of Violets

2 tablespoons expressed   ¼ cup clover or other light
   juice of violets   honey

Mash the violets in gauze to extract the juice, or place in a juicing machine. Mix the two ingredients together by shaking them vigorously in a capped bottle. Use to perfume the breath. When you use the delicate mouthwash, also use a violet perfume so there will be no conflict of scents.

For those who live in the city and do not have access to a meandering patch of violets, it is still possible to have a mouth-freshening liquid which speaks of violets and springtime.

Though the orris root, which gives the scent of violets in the following preparation, comes from the iris plant, it is still a spring-time plant which blooms only shortly after the violet and has much the same delicacy of scent and flavor. Order it from a botanical supply house.

Violet Mouth Freshener

2 tablespoons tincture of orris   2 tablespoons essence of rose
2 cups white vinegar   (see p. 82)
2 tablespoons ethyl alcohol   ⅓ teaspoon oil of peppermint

For tincture of orris root, mix 1 ounce of the powdered root with 2 cups of white vinegar. Place in a glass jar with a tightly fitting lid which excludes all air. Leave in the sunlight for 2 weeks and shake the bottle several times each day. Strain before using.

Mix the 2 tablespoons of tincture of orris root with the essence of rose, alcohol, and peppermint, cap the bottle, and shake well. When you are ready to use it, pour a few drops of the mouth freshener into a little water and rinse the mouth thoroughly. Do not swallow.

Essence of Rose

1 teaspoon natural rose oil   3 tablespoons ethyl alcohol

Shake together in a bottle.

Patience is required for extracting the violet liquid by hand, and it is really a job for a chemist or a juicing machine. But even more difficult is an attempt to obtain oil of violets. So content yourself mostly with eating the violet, both blossom and leaf, and substitute orris root for the extract, as in the following recipe.

Violet Water for Scenting

¾ pound florentine orris root,   1 pint 70 percent ethyl alcohol
    coarsely powdered

Steep for 20 days. Press out the orris root in order to gain the maximum scent. Filter several times and bottle to use as perfume.

REMOVING FACIAL BLOTCHING

A garden which yields cosmetics is a double blessing. Fresh from earth, moist minerals and green and growing plants bring with them a heady combination of beauty possibilities. There is healing in their contents and beauty in their restorative powers. No chemical application can provide the nutrients, energy, and gentle cleansing of parsley, prepared as an infusion to bathe away scaly skin patches of mineral-deficient skin.

In addition, this early spring plant can also help eliminate the red patches of skin that can develop at different times of the year.

Take advantage of this early green and prepare it in liquid form to be used in compresses which will lessen and remove skin blotching which defies conventional treatment of creams and ointments.

Chop a large bunch of washed parsley and place in a glass bowl. Pour a pint of warm distilled or noncarbonated mineral water over it. Allow this to steep, covered, for a full day and night. Strain and dip cloth compresses into the liquid. Apply to the affected areas of the skin. For best results, apply the compresses while lying down. Leave the liquid on to dry after the last compress. Repeat whenever convenient during the day.

CLEOPATRA'S OIL-SCRAPING BATH

For the increasing number of women who find regular bathing devitalizes their skin and brings additional dryness to the tissues, there is an easy and far-from-new remedy at hand. Water may be a contributing factor in dry skin, or the culprit may be an alkaline soap which washes away the acid mantle native to the skin, leaving it dry and chalky.

If you do not wish to change from an alkaline-based soap to an acid-based one which will protect your skin, then your bath water should have a lacing of apple cider vinegar added to it to restore the acid mantle removed by the soap. And no, you won't smell like a pickle. In diluted quantity, the vinegar is hardly noticeable.

Once that practice is established, you might want further insurance in the form of an oil scraping similar to that practiced by early Egyptian and Greek women. First the body was sleeked by massaging golden oil into every pore. Since refined oils were unknown at that time, you can be sure that the body profited from the pureness of the rich oils and that a dry body would thirstily absorb its maximum.

The oils were usually mixed with scent to create a luxurious and pleasant atmosphere while the body was soaking in the nutrients. You could try one oil alone, perhaps sweet almond, olive, sesame seed, or corn oil, or you could combine any or all of these or others, as long as they are polyunsaturated or cold processed oils.

Allow the oil a minimum of 15 minutes to saturate the skin. While your skin is profiting from the penetration of the oils, it would be a good time to spread towels on a slantboard and relax. When you are ready, take a blunt table knife or spatula and carefully scrape the dull side across your oiled body, removing the oil from the knife with a tissue after each stroke.

Do not use force or irritate the skin. The idea is just to remove the top layer of dead scarf skin, without injuring or irritating the underlying tissue. Do not use a sharp knife, kitchen knife, or other dangerous implement.

Cleopatra used a strygil, a blunt-bladed instrument created especially for the scraping treatment. So valued was this oil treatment that strygils were included in burial rites for use after the deceased revived in another world. When the tomb of Queen Hetepheres, mother of Cheops, the pharaoh of the 4th Dynasty (about 3500 B.C.) was opened, included in the toilet articles placed by her side were three of the strygils to ensure her smooth skin in another world.

After gently scraping the skin, taking care to avoid any protrusions, warts, moles, and the like, hop into a warm tub and proceed with your regular bath.

The silkiness of your skin will make this one of your favorite baths, especially after you are forty, for it is then the body oils seem to grow scant and must be replaced with external applications, aided by the daily intake of a polyunsaturated oil in the diet, too.

CHAMOMILE RINSE

Now when the chamomile flower heads are golden and their pungent scent speaks of days when maidens gathered baskets of this exquisite flower for their hair rinse, gather your own supply and give dull, lifeless, or mousy blond hair brightened color. If you haven't a lawn where chamomile has made a soft, fragrant carpet, then be a modern maiden and buy a package of the yellow flower tops from a health food shop or a botanical supply house.

Drop a handful of shredded chamomile flower heads into two cups of cold water. Cover and slowly bring to a boil. Allow the brew to come just under the simmering point for three or four minutes. Remove from the heat and steep for several hours.

After a regular shampoo and regular rinsing pour the strained liquid through the hair over and over again. Catch the chamomile brew in a basin each time. Blot dry, or if possible, do as the medieval maidens did and sit in the sun, allowing it to dry your hair in order to increase the lighter tones. In those days the hazard of sitting outdoors during this treatment was that a knight might come along and sweep you up and away. Unfortunately, that day is long gone, but who knows? Glinting, golden hair can slow down even the fastest driving roadster.

APHRODISIAC FOR APRIL

It seems that almost every culture has contributed some bit of knowledge or quaint custom to the art of aphrodisia. And the search for others continues. Some of the handed-down secrets are very pleasant and might even be effective, if the situation and timing is right.

Foods are classified as amorous if they do more than whet the stomatic appetite. As a matter of fact, medical science really recognizes only two strangely effective aphrodisiacs—Spanish Fly and sap from the yohimbé tree. All other formulas seem to work psychologically by increasing the overall health of the body and improving circulation and performance of the various glands. And imagination.

Why not give one a whirl and try a lovely French springtime aphrodisical violet dish which is as beautiful to see as to taste? What makes it French? Who else but the French would think of putting violets on a custard?

Mix together 4 eggs, beaten, ¼ cup of light honey, ¼ teaspoon salt, 2 cups milk, scalded and cooled to lukewarm, 1 teaspoon arrowroot, and 1 teaspoon of orange flower water. Bake in oiled custard bowl in moderate oven until the custard is firm. Unmold, cool, and cover with fresh violet heads minus the stems.

EXERCISES FOR FLEXIBILITY

The way a woman moves her body says a great deal about her. Does she walk like an automaton, ignoring the asset she could acquire by having a graceful carriage? And the grace doesn't end in appearance only. Underlying a supple, beautiful walk is a comfortable and well-functioning body. To be free of your body, to be able to concentrate on matters of importance and other accomplishments, there must be an ease of body movements.

If you creak and feel a stab of pain when you get up from a seated position, you are likely to go into contortions to avoid the sudden jabs that come with these movements. In defense, you learn to move more slowly, usually with movements which are strictly defensive and therefore suggest an aging body.

Why not rid your body of these minor aches and major annoyances? It is simple to gain a flexible body which will move you through a busy day and allow you to bend, rise, and walk in comfort. The spine determines your degree of suppleness. But in order to gain the degree of mobilization you require, it is necessary after childhood to work the spine daily to prevent stiffness and rigidity from setting in.

One of the easiest and most rewarding exercises for spinal flexibility is so simple and pleasant to perform it can become a morning quickie. It will start you on a day filled with energy.

Stand barefooted, preferably on an uncarpeted floor. This will give you the traction needed to perform the exercise. Place your feet one to one-and-one-half feet apart, with your arms extended at shoulder level to either side. Very slowly, swing the arms, head, and shoulders around to the left as far as they will comfortably go. Keep the feet in position, and without stopping swing the arms back again, this time continuing on to the right. The leading arm will come to rest centered almost directly behind you.

Gradually work up to twenty swings each morning. In addition to flexing the spine, this exercise also slims the waist.

The spinal twist is another excellent way to regain control of your body. These positions will grow easier with each day's practice, and no day should be skipped, for this is a continuing limbering action and requires daily attention in order to be effective.

In a seated position on the floor, extend both legs directly before you. Lift your right foot and place it over your left leg to rest beside the knee. Bring the left arm around to the right side of your right knee and grasp the ankle of your right foot. Be sure to keep your buttocks flat on the floor.

Place your right arm around the waistline of the back of the body with the open palm pointing outward. Twist upper body around to right so that you're looking behind you. Hold the spine upright, and remain in this position for five to ten seconds. Slowly return to your original position by moving your head and shoulders to the front and center. Relax your left arm and remove it from its position. Return the right leg to its prone position outstretched before you.

Relax and then repeat with the other arm and leg.

BREAKFASTS FOR APRIL

Stewed apricots
Granola (recipe on p. 21)
Herbal tea

Orange slices with violets
Poached eggs and wheat germ muffins*
Herbal tea

Grape juice
Millet cereal (recipe on p. 43)
Herbal tea

Stewed prunes
Steamed groats and honey
Herbal tea

Fresh grapefruit
Omclet with chives
Cheese toast
Herbal tea

Applesauce
Mixture of wheat germ, sunflower meal, and oatmeal soaked in
    milk
Herbal tea

Banana slices in fresh orange juice
Omelet filled with violets
Whole grain toast
Herbal tea

LUNCHES FOR APRIL

Watercress soup*
Cheese and apple bowl with greens
Yogurt

Onion Soup*
Mixed green salad bowl
Yogurt

Spring soup*
Cold salmon with mayonnaise and watercress
Yogurt

Grated turnips, carrots, peppers, and radishes
Nut butter sandwiches (recipe on p. 45)
Yogurt

Squash soup
Coleslaw and stuffed eggs
Yogurt

Beet borscht with yogurt*
Parsley, dandelion, and watercress salad

Cheese and vegetable bowl
Cornmeal chapaties (recipe on p. 23)
Yogurt

DINNERS FOR APRIL

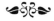

Steamed fish with parsley and chives
Broiled tomatoes
Pilaf

Pecan loaf
Broccoli in lemon sauce
Steamed shredded beets

Sautéed brains
Baked potato
Turnip greens

Broiled chicken
Brown rice cooked in broth
Leafy green vegetable

Broiled liver
Cauliflower
Peas

Cheese soufflé
Fiddle-neck fern or fresh peas

Soybean burgers*
Stewed tomatoes
String beans

RECIPES FOR APRIL

Wheat Germ Muffins

¾ cup milk
2 eggs
3 tablespoons honey
3 tablespoons oil

1 cup wheat germ
1 cup whole wheat flour
4 teaspoons baking powder
½ teaspoon sea salt

Blend liquids together and beat in wheat germ. Sift other dry ingredients together and add to the first mixture, beating thoroughly.
Pour into oiled muffin tins and bake for 25 minutes at 400 degrees.

Watercress Soup

3 potatoes, sliced
4 cups bouillon
2 cups watercress

sea salt to taste
1 cup milk
1 teaspoon salad oil

Cook potatoes in bouillon until barely soft. Add the watercress and
salt and cook for 3 or 4 minutes more. Place in blender with
milk and oil and blend smooth. Serve with chopped fresh watercress on top.

Spring Soup

½ cup chopped carrot
½ cup chopped onion
½ cup chopped celery
½ cup fresh dandelion leaves

arrowroot
4 cups chicken stock
1 tablespoon oil
sea salt

Cook vegetables in stock until soft. Strain and put vegetables aside. Mix enough arrowroot with water to form a thin paste and stir slowly into the stock along with the oil. Cook until thickened. Return vegetables to soup and cook until heated. Season to taste with sea salt.

Beet Borscht with Yogurt

3 beets, shredded
4 cups meat stock

1 lemon
sea salt

Cook beets in stock until tender. Place in blender with juice of the lemon and 1 tablespoon of grated lemon rind. Add salt and yogurt and blend to a smooth consistency. Serve with a dab of yogurt on top.

Onion Soup

2 cups thinly sliced onions
2 tablespoons sweet butter
1 tablespoon arrowroot
4 cups water

2 cups consommé
¼ cup heated milk
¼ pound grated Swiss cheese
2 tablespoons melted butter

Cook onions and 2 tablespoons of hard butter in heavy skillet until golden brown. Add arrowroot to 1 cup of water and set aside. Pour consommé and 3 cups of water over the onions in the skillet and bring to a boil, stirring constantly. Simmer for 15 minutes and add the milk. Slowly stir in the arrowroot mixture and continue cooking until slightly thickened. Pour into ovenproof bowl and sprinkle with the grated cheese which has been mixed with the melted butter. Brown quickly under the broiler and serve.

Soybean Burgers

1 cup soybeans, cooked and
    mashed
1 egg, beaten
4 tablespoons wheat germ

yogurt to moisten
1 tablespoon minced onion
1 tablespoon minced celery

Mix together and form into flat patties and bake on hot griddle.

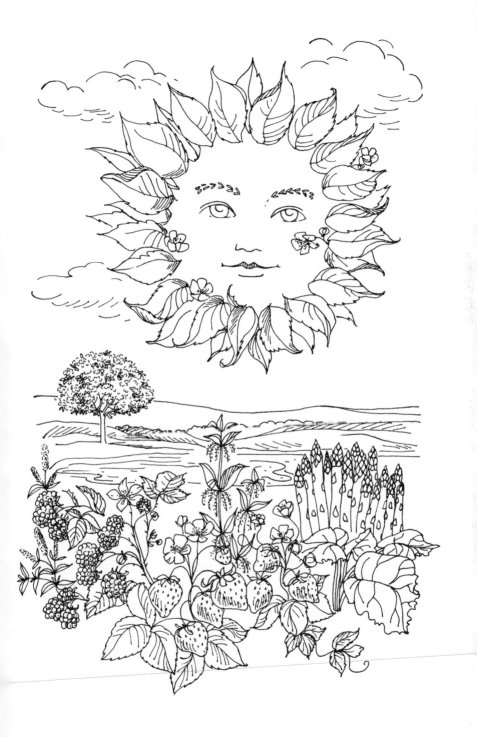

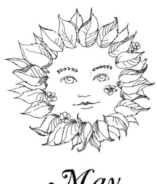

May

It's like the birthday of the world,
When earth was born in bloom;
The light is made of many dyes,
The air is all perfume:
There's crimson buds, and white and
blue,
The very rainbow showers
Have turned to blossoms where they fell
And sown the earth with flowers.

> *Thomas Hood: "Song"*

The Goddess of Growth and Increase, Maia, gave her name to this dazzling month. The Dutch referred to it as the Blossoming Month, while the French calendar acknowledged it as The Time of Flowers.

And true enough. There are the first berries on the vine, new shoots of growth on bush and tree, and according to where you live in the world, flowers of every scent and color to eat, to wear, and to use for heady lotions and potions. The Saxons, less romantic and more realistic, called this month Thrice Milked because the cows, luxuriating in new green fodder, could be milked three times a day. In honor of that tradition, one could loll in a lovely milk bath, realizing there is splendor in this, too. Or, if you prefer, soak your thirsty body skin in a strengthening and absorbable bath of fruit leaves taken from newly sprouted berry vines.

Has there ever been a time when life was not present and renewing itself? Man's earliest records speak of growth and change and betterment. And the awe-inspiring fact of life itself promises this eternal renewal. Does spring not follow winter, and when winter tucks in the last leaf and covers all sleeping nature, is it indeed gone, or isn't this merely a renewal process which is going on? Nature falls back and prepares, but rises again and again and again, as promised with the last snowflake, and the first leaf.

How can one doubt the resurgence of life when it has gone on, centuries beyond count, never disappearing, only changing in form. The body joins in this re-creation, this plan of life, encouraging growth, providing a generous nature to make it possible.

The early festival of the Druids with their rituals in praise and thanksgiving of the life-bringing summer months continues in our own picnic excursions, May Day parties, and Strawberry Festivals. We give primitive recognition, dressed in modern style, to our source of sustenance and renewal.

Green growth is upon the land this month, and the hungry body reaches for the first garden things, no less than the deer nibbles eagerly at the first birch buds after a long winter. All living things turn to the warming sun, and those hungry for physical renewal reach for herb and flower, for plant and vine.

With seeming awareness that spring housecleaning is beneficial to the body, nature produces two of the finest natural aperients known. While May flowers bloom above them, asparagus tips thrust fleshy, sweet-tasting, helmeted buds skyward and await only cutting to add a powerhouse of vitamins and minerals to the diet. And this nourishing spring vegetable also sweeps out accumulated debris from the cluttered body.

Eaten raw, the tips and stems of asparagus help to cleanse the blood supply and wash away impurities, giving a glow to the sallow and wan face that shows deprivation of the nutrients found in this vegetable.

Rhubarb also adds its tonic action to the ritual of spring. Using small quantities of the stems of this rosy fruit cooked with honey increases the regularity so essential to an unblemished complexion. No beauty can exist when impurities and toxins remain in a sluggish, malfunctioning body.

So accept the gifts of spring. Scout out the first offerings in garden or market. Eat them frequently, and remember this was the way the sturdy early American maintained his health, after winter privation, and how these health practices led to the appellation "American Beauty" for lovely, pink-cheeked women of an earlier day. Join them in practice, and watch your own skin come alive. Check your diet daily to see how many really fresh, unfrozen, uncanned, unprocessed foods are on your plate.

TO GATHER AND CLARIFIE MAY DEW

When there hath fallen no raine the night before, then with a cleane and large sponge, the next morning, you may gather the same from sweet herbs, grasse or corne: straine your dew, and expose it to the Sun in glasses covered with papers or parchments prickt full of holes; straine it often, continuing it in the Sun, and in an hot place, till the same grow white and cleare, which will require the best part of the Summer.

Some commend May-dew, gathered from Fennell and Celandine to be most excellent for sore eyes: and some commend the same (prepared as before) above Rose-water for preserving of fruits, flowers, etc.

Ram's Little Dadoen, 1606

Medieval stories always describe the maiden as being of delicate countenance. According to the tales of that day, her skin was like a rose petal, her cheeks were faintly tinged with pink, and she was a veritable cameo of perfection. Old tapestries and woodcuts show these ethereal maidens out gathering herbs to make potions which supposedly rendered them all fair and exquisite. And from that period comes these instructions for gathering May dew, which was supposed to soften, whiten, lighten, and produce some or all of this delicate beauty. For fun and possible profit, why not try this old recipe, if you live in an area away from the modern hazards of automobile fumes.

THE MEANINGFUL BATH

Beauty bathing is one of the most pleasant ways to treat a body which is exhausted, out of tone, or in need of general stimulation. According to the condition of your body, you can revive it with an herbal solution, remove coarsened and dead tissue with a friction rub of sea salt, or nourish it with a creamy oatmeal liquid or bran lotion which returns hormones and oils to a depleted skin.

Bathing can invigorate, restore skin beauty, and produce serenity, and for more than two thousand years these qualities have been sought out in various baths. Beauty spas in Europe are popular resorts which have never lost favor. Even in America, mineral water baths were once in favor at such spas as Saratoga Springs, N.Y., Greenbrier, W. Va., and Hot Springs, Ark.

Health spas located near a natural source of beneficial mineral waters offer mineral-rich baths which can help expand the capillaries and improve circulation, and in this manner increase body beauty through greater blood flow. One resort in Germany offers a thermal bath, particularly suited for restorative bathing. Its waters have a sodium-magnesium-hydrogen-carbonate content charged with carbon dioxide in combined as well as disassociated form.

In addition, there are herbal baths and mud baths. The value of the latter lies in the concentrated minerals found in the lava-based mud.

The Soviet Union, too, has delved in recent times into the practice of balneology, or the use of water to cure and prevent illness. Scientists there believe that the best way to do this is to stimulate the body's own resistant and defensive forces.

The American Indians knew the value of natural hot springs, and carried ailing people by litter to these places for restorative baths, probably bouncing the life out of them by the time they got there. Apparently, however, they thought it was worth it.

While the mineral waters available in spas around the world sound attractive and seductively pleasant, there are solutions you can produce in your own home which will do much to treat and pamper the body and produce a fine skin tissue, a stronger and more youthful vigor, and at the same time, help to create the serenity and tranquillity that allows you to greet each day with joy and to retire each night in peace.

Summertime, with its riot of growth in field and garden, offers a wealth of choice for youthifying baths. The clever woman sows specific plants for special needs, and reaps a harvest of beauty for her bath. Though not everyone has access to a garden, it is still possible to gather the necessary materials for these beauty baths.

Field and roadside grow magnificent "weeds." Learning to identify wild herbs is a delight in itself. These unsprayed crops grow largely unnoticed, enriching only the banks and hummocks or plains upon which they grow. Catch up a basket and clippers and go journeying through the woodlands and open areas in search of this perpetual beauty supply. Carry gloves in order to protect yourself against poison ivy and stinging nettle—although the nettle offers an array of body benefits for one careful enough to avoid direct contact with it.

Snip it off with shears, never touching the plant or leaves with your bare hands as long as it is fresh, rather than dried. Like many other herbs, stinging nettle is dried and crumbled before steeping in an infusion, or tea, to produce a potent liquid which will benefit the body. Once the nettle plant is dried, it is safe to touch, for the formic acid that creates blisters disappears.

Gather peppermint, comfrey, sage, rosemary, and verbena for your bath. Add lemon balm, thyme, and dill. These dried herbs can be used either singly or mixed into a potpourri, according to your own needs. An attractive way to store and enjoy herbs for beauty bathing is in a group of apothecary jars lining a shelf. Into each one place the completely dried plants or petals and cover it tightly with a lid. Then, when you are preparing your bath, go "shopping" in front of your storage jars and decide whether you want a stimulating, relaxing, soothing, or strengthening bath, and select your mixture accordingly.

Alongside your jars you might want to include small bottles of perfumed oils, to be used for a sense of pleasure, which certainly is desirable in any beauty bathing. But do not mix the oils with the herbs, for the plants have a much more delicate perfume and their scent would be overcome by the stronger oils. Rather, reserve the concentrated oils to mix with oatmeal, bran, or vegetable oil baths.

Perhaps you would also like some small bath bags which take only a moment to fill and use. Dried or fresh herbs can go into the cotton bags, which are hung around the bathtub faucet so the water runs through and releases the scents and oils in the dried petals and leaves.

Rosemary's aromatic qualities have endeared it to centuries of luxury bathers, and countless generations have praised its use. Also called "Dew of the Sea," this Biblical plant offers its cure-all effectiveness to most parts of the world. You can find baskets of it in shops on islands off the coast of Greece or see it flourishing in American gardens and treasured in England.

The camphorated quality of rosemary's oil makes it especially valuable to those with skin troubles. Healing, soothing, and medicinal, rosemary's scent and oil have haunted their way through time. Poets have extolled its value and credited it with a range of benefits which boggle the mind. Only use the astringent oil and you will feel uplifted by its pungent scent.

In the French language of flowers, rosemary is said to rekindle lost energy. When it is placed under a pillow, herbal belief says it is supposed to replace nightmares with sweet dreams. This plant seems to have captivated the world in earlier times, and wherever it was seen, it was considered a good omen. As a stimulator for appetites, a lotion for a weakened body, and a wash for problem hair, there seemed no better application than either leaf, stem, or flower of the valued rosemary.

There are other herbs of renown, too. An infusion of valerian root has long been used as a calming additive to bath water in Europe. In the field of pharmacopeia, it is used as a sedative. Those with a nervous disposition might well profit from brewing up a pint or so of this pretty plant and adding it to a tub of warm water. With its rich silica content, balsamic resin, minerals, and valerianin, it seems to act upon jangled nerves to produce calm and a desire to sleep.

Since the human skin should, under healthy conditions, eliminate around 30 percent of inner wastes, it is necessary to keep the millions of minuscule pores open to carry out this work. If the body has been casually bathed with a brief shower and a bar of soap, you can almost be assured you have not promoted your own health and comfort. Clogging overworked pores with a layer of soap that isn't properly rinsed away is the same as applying a film barrier to the skin.

Scented vinegar is a delightful way to remove alkaline soap deposits from the skin and restore its natural acid mantle. One such formula, more than one hundred years old, works just as well today as it did when the mixture was poured into a galvanized tub of well water that had been heated on a wood burning stove. And the famous Harriet Hubbard Ayer, who used the formula to help make her the noted beauty and beautician of her day, left the instructions for future generations, bless her.

Bruise 1 pint of ripe strawberries (not half ripe, but soft, sweetly scented fully ripe berries). Add to 1 pint of white vinegar and let stand for 24 hours. Press the mixture through cotton or linen and squeeze out all the juice. Add 8 ounces of rose water (which you can purchase in some gourmet shops, or through a pharmacist, or make yourself).

Or you can use elderflower water or other scented flower water. Add 1 cup of the solution to a half filled tub of warm water and luxuriate. This stimulating and slightly astringent lotion can also be used on the hands and face outside the bath.

Whether you try a strawberry, rosemary, blackberry, or vinegar bath, each should be meaningful and more than a splash through the tub or shower. May is the month of renewal, and there is no better way to participate in nature's process than to refresh and reinvigorate your tired winter body and skin. So bathe your body and let it breathe!

BLACKBERRY BATH FOR MAY

Bathe away the winter's humors, herbalists have advised, both internally and externally. With the early offerings of springtime gardens and fields coming alive with jewel leaves of vigorous plants, this is the time to tone and treat a body grown pallid from long months of heavy clothes and the laziness of indoor living.

Blackberry vines are an excellent source of iron to help create red blood so needed by a body renewing itself. The tannin in the leaves makes this an astringent and therefore valuable in treating skin problems.

Preparation for your blackberry leaf bath must be done in advance. Pick the young leaves early in the springtime and dry them well. This can be done in a very low oven, or simply by using the usual herb drying process.

When you are ready to have your blackberry leaf bath, crumble a pint of the dried leaves into 3 quarts of boiling water. Do not cook the leaves, but rather remove the pot from the heat and steep for 10 minutes before straining into half a tub of warm water. Relax in the bath for 15 to 20 minutes, allowing the body to absorb the curative qualities that make the blackberry leaf a skin healer and refresher. For the best results, this should be taken 3 times a week.

BLACKBERRY PACK FOR THE FACE

Follow up the blackberry bath with a facial pack of blackberry leaves. They have a cleansing, astringent action.

Gather 2 or 3 handfuls of young green leaves and mince them finely before tossing into a cup of boiling water. Stew gently a few minutes until they are soft and mushy. Gather them together in a double cheesecloth covering, lie down, and press the pack upon your face. Again, the slantboard is beneficial here, as with its use the blood comes more quickly to the facial area and assists the application in penetrating. Relax with the leaves covering the face for 15 minutes. Rinse away the residue without using soap, and blot the skin. If your skin is dry, apply a thin film of salad oil afterward.

BLACKBERRY RINSE FOR OILY HAIR

Treasured by country people accustomed to taking care of their cosmetic problems by turning to nature, the blackberry bush yields an especially fine rinse for hair which requires shampooing too frequently.

Rather than stripping your hair of its oils by too-frequent dousings with suds, you might like to try an old-fashioned folk remedy for excessive scalp oil. After your regular shampoo, rinse the hair thoroughly, blot dry, and then, as a final and usually quite effective rinse, pour a solution made from blackberry leaves over your hair. Catch the water in a basin and repeat the rinsing process three or four times.

Chop 2 cups of fresh young blackberry leaves and toss them into 2 cups of boiling water in an enamel, glass, or stainless steel pot. Simmer, with a lid on, for 5 minutes. Remove from the heat and steep for 10 minutes. Strain and allow the liquid to become lukewarm before using.

LETTUCE LOTION

Look around you in this awakening month and take advantage of everything that is fresh and growing to aid your complexion. Create a skin as flawless and smooth as it was years ago by giving it frequent attention. You will be rewarded with a tightened skin and a pearly translucent appearance.

Try a lettuce lotion facial and apply it daily, letting the rich vitamins and minerals strengthen and build up skin tissue. Antonius Musa, physician to Emperor Augustus, was an early organic doctor, since he prescribed lettuce as a health food, which indeed it is. And a beauty food, too. That is, as long as it is a sturdy type of lettuce rather than the iceberg variety which has little if any nourishment in it. So use the young garden lettuce in both your diet and complexion care, and watch the bloom emerge in your cheeks.

Drop a handful of green lettuce leaves into an enamel or glass pot and cover with boiling water. Cover and simmer for ½ hour. Mash the leaves in the water or place both liquid and leaves in the blender and liquefy. Strain into a clean jar and beat in a few drops of tincture of benzoin. Keep refrigerated, and use as a facial lotion.

HERBAL TOOTHPOWDER

One of the more pleasant discoveries in the lives of many people is that one can be unchained from the toothpowder and toothpaste syndrome. The search for a whiter, tastier, foamier, cavity-chasing toothpaste which spins from a tube can really become a preoccupation as you drift from one highly marketed item to another.

Try making your own tooth cleanser and give up all doubts of what cleanses best. Even before the time when sweet gum brushes served both as cleanser and toothpaste, herbs were used to both sweeten and cleanse the mouth. And in today's attempt to avoid the sometimes-questionable ingredients in toothpastes and powders, it is simple enough to turn to home concoctions for effective cleansing preparations. Try this herbal mixture for removing stains and brightening the teeth.

Sage and Salt Toothpowder

Use equal quantities, perhaps ¼ cup each, of salt and sage leaves. Rub them together in a mortar and pestle until they blend. Sprinkle with water to give adhesion and bake in a shallow pan in a moderate oven until thoroughly dry. Grind again with the mortar and pestle into a powder.

STRENGTHENING THE FINGERNAILS

Summer's brilliance of colors depends in part on May planting in most areas around North America. And while planting seeds can be an enriching occupation with the two immediate benefits of serenity of mind and body toning, digging into the soil can take its toll from unprotected hands and fingernails. Soft, easily damaged fingernails sometimes cannot even come through gloved gardening without a snag, tear, or torn-off section. But this is not too difficult to avoid if you take the time to strengthen your nails before the season gets under way.

One method used to reinforce fingernails is a warm olive oil bath. Heat ½ cup of oil in a glass container. Every other day, submerge the nails for 10 minutes; remove from the oil and blot dry. It may take a few weeks to notice improvement, but eventually your nails will grow firmer.

Another nail aid calls for making a fingerbath of the herb horsetail. The silica content of this venerable plant makes it valuable in the treatment of many areas of the body, as long as one is knowledgeable about its medicinal and antiseptic qualities.

For an herbal nail strengthener, chop ¼ cup of horsetail and add to 1 cup of water. Simmer for 5 minutes and steep, covered, for several hours. Strain and use in the same manner as the oil bath—by submerging the fingertips into the liquid for 10 minutes every other day until the nails grow stronger.

DEEP PORE CLEANSER

Soap, according to its composition, and water can be good cleansing agents for oily or even normal skins. Used with a complexion brush, natural sponge, or even a sturdy face cloth, the gentle rubbing action and lather can dissolve and float away makeup, grime, and other debris. But there is another facial cleanser which is so effective it can remove additional grime even after a thorough scrubbing with soap and water.

Milk and oil, beaten together thoroughly, form one of the finest skin cleansers available. And it is yours for pennies. But it must be prepared daily or kept refrigerated, and it cannot be used after its freshness is gone. Therefore, prepare it in small quantities, and if you see it lasts too long, cut down the original recipe to suit your own needs. With this cleanser, you need soft, absorbent cotton balls. Ordinary tissues just won't do, for they become too harsh when dipped into the mixture.

Sesame Seed Cleanser

Mix 1 teaspoon of sesame seed oil with 2 tablespoons of milk and shake together vigorously to homogenize. Using small cotton balls, dip into the liquid and rub well into the skin in a circular motion. Change pads often as you lift makeup or grime from your face. Rinse in warm, then cool, water and blot dry.

FLABBY SKIN LOTION

While practicing exercises to tighten loose flesh and return skin tone to your body, lend additional help in every way possible by applying strengthening, nourishing, and stimulating natural foods and products to the weakened areas.

The general rule for beauty calls for constant and unstinting attention to those areas that can be referred to as trouble spots. The upper part of the arm is such an area. The lotion here helps in returning tone to the skin through a combined value as an astringent and the massage that accompanies it.

Place 1 cucumber in the blender and reduce to a pulp. (Use the peel, unless it is waxed or heavily coated with oil.) Strain through gauze to produce 4 tablespoons of juice. Beat in 3 teaspoons of tincture of benzoin, which serves to firm the flesh, and add half a cup of water. Bottle and refrigerate until ready to use. Gently massage into the troubled area twice a day, preferably morning and night.

If you don't have a blender, chop the cucumber finely and squeeze through gauze to produce the juice, then proceed with the formula.

SAGE HAIR TONIC AND COLORANT

It is not easy to avoid chemical hair dyes after forty and, for some, even before, when the natural hair coloring begins to fade and gray streaks appear. Some herbs will conceal the gray that will eventually become the predominant non-color. Mixtures of black tea, rosemary, walnut hulls, or just a strong sage tea will sometimes help color graying hair.

An old recipe for darkening hair suggests mixing 2 tablespoons each of dried sage and black tea or, if that is not available, regular tea. Place these ingredients in the top of a double boiler and pour 2 cups of boiling water over the mixture. Cover and simmer for an hour.

Steep until cold, strain, and pour off enough each day to saturate the roots of the hair. Massage in with a cotton ball and work upward to cover every strand. Repeat this every day until you have the color you want, then try applying it every other night, or as frequently as is required to maintain the color.

BUTTERMILK WASH

Buttermilk wash contains magic in its two ingredients, and they are no more than simple foods. We all know the wonders of oatmeal—how it bleaches, cleans, softens, and nourishes. Add to that the stimulating qualities of buttermilk and you have an astringent wash which is helpful for oily skin and sallow complexions.

Mix enough finely ground or powdered oatmeal with enough buttermilk to form a thickened liquid or thin paste. It must be very easy to spread. Rub this gently onto the face and neck and give it time to dry. Remove by using a damp washcloth and rubbing gently in an upward circular motion until you have covered the entire face and neck.

Keep rinsing out the washcloth and wring it as dry as possible each time. Splash an apple cider vinegar and water solution over your face as a last rinse and blot it dry.

CASBAH MINT FOR A MAY APHRODISIAC

Arabs have always prized hot mint tea for its stimulating qualities, no matter what the season. Wherever you go in the Csabah in Tangiers, you'll find little café tables supporting the elbows of robed Romeos bent forward over steaming glasses of tea.

Hot, sweet, and pungent from the crushed mint leaves, Casbah tea almost immediately comforts the body. Perhaps arousal comes next, but comfort alone is great. To be relaxed is conducive to love, so you might well count this as an important aphrodisiac. The Arabs do.

And more than 100 million Arabs couldn't be wrong. They sip their hot minted tea and then fold up their tents and weave, wraith-like, through the winding streets of the Casbah into those shady enclosed compounds wherein await equally swathed and tented ladies. Drinking their own mint tea.

So brew a pot of sweet mint tea. Crush the mint, place it in the bottom of a cup or glass, and pour scalding, honey-sweetened tea over the fragrant herb; stir. And then fold up your tent.

SHOULDERS AND ARMS

As the days grow warmer, you begin to shed layers of clothing like a caterpillar. Now it is the time for short-sleeved and sleeveless dresses and blouses. Come spring, however, you may be appalled at the loss of tone in the upper region of the body. Arms you had believed firm and smooth can show slack flesh when framed by a sleeveless blouse or halter.

What to do? Go back to long sleeves and hide the condition? Not at all. Get to work today and develop firm-fleshed, pretty arms which complement your body. Besides, the exercises will bring additional stimulation which will add to your zest for living.

Sometimes the shock of seeing skin-tone loss can actually work as a therapeutic device for a woman. If she reacts by resolving to overcome her problem, she can revitalize her whole body, and in doing this, develop greater scope which will extend to other areas of living. The well-exercised body does not show the wear and tear of years the way the neglected one does. And the neglected body can also be an indication that a woman is not actually fulfilling herself in all the ways she can.

ARM EXERCISES

The following movements are aimed at firming the upper-arm area, one of the first places that falls slack and indicates atrophy. Daily exercise with the upper arms can give thrilling results as you notice the flesh firming and your arm returning to an attractive condition.

Stand upright, with the head centered and the chin parallel to the floor. Extend your arms before you with the palms up. Taking a deep breath, drop the right arm down close to the body and, without stopping motion, continue backward, up, and around again to the starting position.

Repeat this movement with the left arm, always returning to a palm-up position. Practice only two or three times the first day, and if comfortable, work up to a half dozen times.

For another helpful exercise, stand upright and extend both arms out from the shoulders. Hold your arm as though you were about to slap an oncoming ball. Your elbow will be slightly bent as you spread your fingers and hand, with the palm facing the oncoming ball.

Slowly, with fingers spread, sweep inward toward the chest, touching it lightly before slowly swinging out again. Repeat the movement with the left arm. Alternate the right and left arm. To test the effectiveness of this marvelous arm exercise, reach over and touch the underarm area of the right or left arm while the other is performing. If you have not tensed your hand enough, a slackness will remain in the underarm area.

An exercise taught in beauty spas around the world seems to be universal in presentation. One will come across it in a California health resort, on a beauty farm in Pennsylvania, and in an elegant spa in Switzerland. It is simple enough to perform and produces good results if practiced daily.

Standing upright, extend the arms directly out from the shoulders to each side. Start rotating the hands from relaxed wrists. Let the hands create a small circle, with as little movement or assistance from the arms as possible. In this manner, the pull on the underarm area is more concentrated. Reverse the position and rotate the wrists in the opposite direction.

Now, drop both arms and repeat the hand rotation with the arms hanging by the sides, but not touching the body. Reverse positions and repeat.

BREAKFASTS FOR MAY

Fresh minted orange slices
Rice omelet*
Herbal tea

Cranberry juice
Muesli with currants
Herbal tea

Stewed apricots
Cheese toast
Herbal tea

Stewed rhubarb and honey
Poached egg
Wheat germ muffins (recipe on p. 92)
Herbal tea

Broiled bananas
Oatmeal with wheat germ and sesame seed
Herbal tea

Applesauce with rhubarb
Brown rice flour pancakes (recipe on p. 21)
Herbal tea

Prunes and lemon slices cooked together
Kasha (buckwheat)*
Herbal tea

LUNCHES FOR MAY

Spring drink*
Asparagus and cheese on whole wheat toast
Green salad
Yogurt

Carrot and celery juice
Portuguese sardines and coleslaw
Yogurt

Fresh green pea soup*
Nut butter sandwiches (recipe on p. 45)
Yogurt

Whole potato soup (recipe on p. 22)
Toasted cheese sandwiches
Yogurt

Carrot soup*
Avocado, grape, and banana salad
Yogurt

Cauliflower soup*
Shredded green cabbage, apple, and radishes
Yogurt

Puree of string bean soup (recipe on p. 47)
Shredded carrots, beets, and green pepper salad
Yogurt

DINNERS FOR MAY

᭣᭟᭢

Broiled fish
Potatoes steamed in jackets, with parsley and oil dressing
Mustard greens

Nutburgers*
Acorn squash
Spinach and onion salad

Chicken baked in wheat germ
Baked potato
Shredded cooked beets

Stuffed peppers (recipe on p. 71)
Herbed rice
Broccoli

Chicken livers en brochette with fresh pineapple
Green noodles with lemon and vegetable oil
Asparagus

Combination ground heart and beef
Potatoes steamed in jackets
Chard or steamed cabbage

Soy-rice bake*
Steamed cabbage
Shredded steamed beets

RECIPES FOR MAY

Rice Omelet

3 eggs
1 cup cooked brown rice
1 tablespoon melted butter

1 cup milk
seasoning

Beat eggs to a lemony color and blend into the warm rice. Add the melted butter. Blend in the heated milk and seasonings and pour into a buttered omelet pan, to bake at 400 degrees in a hot oven. After omelet has set completely, fold in half and allow top to brown.

Kasha

3 cups milk or water
½ cup buckwheat groats

salt and butter to season

Bring the liquid to a boil and slowly stir in the groats, salt, and butter. Simmer for 10 minutes. Serve hot with milk and honey.

Spring Drink

1 cup fresh fruit juice—orange, pineapple, or other
1 cup fresh green leaves— parsley, mint, watercress, etc.
1 chopped apple

Liquefy in the blender.

Fresh Green Pea Soup

Cook 1 cup of freshly shelled green peas for 4 minutes, or just until barely tender, with 2 chicken bouillon cubes in just enough water to prevent scorching. In a blender add the soup to 1 teaspoon of minced onion, and 2 cups of milk, and blend on high speed until smooth. Season with a pinch of mace and serve cold.

Carrot Soup

Cook 1 cup of chopped carrots and 1 cup of potatoes in a small amount of water. When barely tender, add enough hot milk to form a thick soup and mix in blender. Season with celery salt and whir in 1 tablespoon of vegetable or nut oil. Serve hot.

Cauliflower Soup

Cook 1 cup of cauliflower in a small amount of water with a pinch of sea salt. Add $\frac{1}{4}$ cup minced parsley and 1 teaspoon of minced green onion and enough hot milk to make a thick soup. In blender, mix until smooth and serve hot.

Nutburgers

2 cups cooked brown rice	¼ cup minced parsley
1 beaten egg	2 teaspoons lemon juice
½ cup chopped walnuts	1 tablespoon vegetable oil

Mix ingredients together. Make small-sized patties. Bake on hot griddle and serve immediately.

Soy-Rice Bake

2 cups cooked mashed soy-beans	¼ cup minced onion
1 cup cooked brown rice	¼ cup minced celery
½ cup ground nutmeats	1 beaten egg
1 bouillon cube dissolved in 2 tablespoons water	2 tablespoons oil
	½ crushed whole wheat cracker crumbs

Mix together and bake in an oiled casserole at 350 degrees for 1 hour. Serve with tomato sauce.

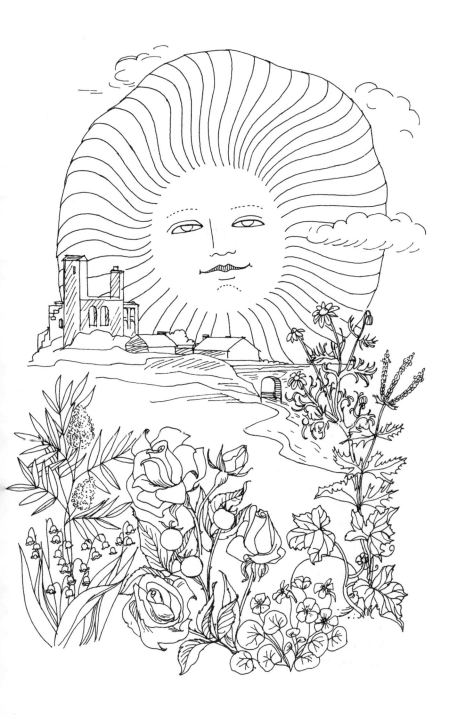

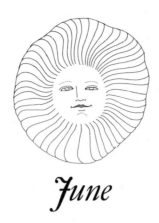

June

And what is so rare as a day in June?
Then, if ever, come perfect days;
Then heaven tries the earth if it be in
tune,
And over it softly her warm ear lays.

James Russell Lowell:
"Vision of Sir Launfal"

Named from the Roman Junius, suggesting young or youthful, this month carries its name well. The Dutch called it Summer Month and the Saxons Dry Month and Joy Time. In the French calendar it was known as Meadow Month, and June marriages are considered lucky.

And why not? The sun's in the sky, the sky is blue, and growth is everywhere. You can live free and easy and plan for long, summery days in which to renew your acquaintance with the land. There is a wealth of lovely, fresh things to tempt the body and cure it, to revive the complexion, and you can take in long breaths of sweet-smelling scents, flung out in abandon by a generous nature.

You can choose at will the scented teas of serenity—lemon balm, mint, verbena, or raspberry. And splash the nectared honey dew upon a thirsty skin to freshen and cool it, while lolling in a tub of some scented flower brew. Then there are strawberry facials to bleach, smooth, and clear, and to pop into the mouth just for sensual joy. These are the perfect days.

HERB PILLOW FOR JUNE

Lack of sleep can do ruinous damage to your face and disposition. Sometimes, when insomnia is simply a matter of a restless mind, an old-fashioned and delightful herb pillow can be very soothing.

For centuries before there were sleeping pills, herbs were used to calm anxiety. And sleep brought on by these simple natural products leaves you far more refreshed in the morning than one induced by barbiturates.

Hops in a pillow is an ancient and reliable means of drifting off to sleep. But since this vine is generally not cultivated except for commercial use in breweries, it is rather difficult to obtain, though it once grew in every colonial garden. In any event, you can substitute other effective herbs. One soothing mixture, a favorite of Charles II's wife, calls for 1 quart of rose petals which have been dried in an airy room away from strong sunlight. A flat pan or oblong basket is best for drying. Sift through the petals every day to speed the process.

When the petals are completely dry, add 1 cupful each of dried rosemary leaves, thyme, and lavender. Grate the dried rind of 1 orange and add 2 teaspoons of powdered cloves. Mix together well and place in 4 x 6 squares of silk or cotton. Place them under your regular pillow for a good night's sleep and pleasant dreams.

FOOT CARE FOR JUNE

The same summer weather that makes roses bloom and color reappear on skin too long deprived of sun brings with it the need for better foot care. Our feet require occasional freedom from their prison of hosiery and shoes in order to avoid some of the more common foot ailments and diseases.

Why not launch a new program of foot care and plan to increase your comfort by giving a little summer care to these often-neglected members? Have a lawn? Then walk on it barefooted. Recapture the satin-green grass memory as you mow, garden, or simply take a barefooted walk around your grounds. Even a small patch of green will suffice for this pleasant occupation. And you can always head for the park and shed your shoes there for an occasional stroll.

You will be helping your feet to better health with these simple practices. If you can't find a patch of lawn anywhere and a park isn't available, remove your shoes for some portion of the day and walk barefoot on the carpeting or floor in your own home. Foot freedom for at least part of the day is vital for the best foot health.

Fatigued, aching feet can also know almost instant rejuvenation and comfort from an old-fashioned foot bath containing tincture of arnica. The arnica plant grows lustily in the West, and was a cherished American Indian remedy for relieving aching muscles and exhausted limbs long before the white man came and helped himself to it. Available from a pharmacy as a tincture, this official drug plant can also be ordered in dried-flower form from botanical supply houses. For ease of preparation, the tincture, or concentrate of the plant, would perhaps be best. A few drops mixed into a small basin of warm water will prove a beneficial stimulator to perspiring and aching summer feet. Keep the feet immersed in the basin for thirty minutes. Then dry them with sturdy toweling, removing every bit of moisture and paying special attention to the areas between the toes, for it is here that infections easily begin in moist skin.

For greater softness, rub a small amount of sweet almond oil into the well-dried skin in upward movements from the toes toward the ankles. Blot away any excess oil.

HERBAL TEAS FOR SERENITY

For centuries, herbs have been used to good benefit for allaying nervousness. Through use over ever so many generations, certain plants have been established as having specific benefits, and their effectiveness has been authenticated by herbalists' handbooks and family recipes.

Instead of reaching for a tranquilizer when life grows hectic and your nerves are shattered, try a cup of beauty tea. This would be an herb drink, selected for the specific quality you need. Sip a cup of it two or three times a day. Not only will you be able to forego the tranquilizer, but the qualities in the herb will soothe and calm and help internally in various beneficial ways.

Herbs have a multitude of uses. In addition to serving as a beverage, they have been used by man for magic, cosmetics (which can be a form of magic when they work), medicine, cooking, and disguising odors, among others. But to soothe tension and to ease and relax a wrinkled brow, try a cup of herb tea.

In Biblical times and before, herbs brought peace and comfort to the harried mind and pained body. There was never a question as to the efficacy of herbs for any and all ailments in earlier days.

Even broken bones were declared helped and mended by applying Eupatorium Agrimony, or boneset. Though in origin its name comes from Mithridates, called Eupator, or he of noble fathers, its reputation as a mender of broken bones has brought it down through the ages simply as boneset.

As far as relating herbal teas to beauty, any food or liquid which brings calm and tranquillity can be considered a beauty treatment. Nature and wisdom always say the same, according to Juvenal, the Roman poet. To be calm, to be placid, is to be at one with nature. There can be no beauty when there are tightly compressed lips, mouths pulled into a taut line, or a harried mind and distraught body.

The scent alone of a cup of herbal tea can bring a feeling of pleasure and hence relaxation to the ragged mind. In addition, there are digestive properties in some plants which make them invaluable. For good digestion is vital to a good disposition and a good complexion.

MINT TEA

Mint tea is an excellent stimulant to digestion, and acts also as a tonic. This is an enjoyable way to end a meal and at the same time aid in the digestive processes. One of the more widely used herbs, mint comes in some forty varieties, including peppermint, woolymint, lemon, and spearmint.

Mint lingers in fragrance and memory, much like the legend of its origin. Taking its name from Minthe, beloved of Pluto, this lovely, trailing plant with lilac-shadowed color was the result of the jealousy of Pluto's wife, Prosperine, who transformed the nymph into an eternally wandering vine.

The nymph-turned-herb certainly has wandered far. Mint is a popular drink around the world, lauded for the many and varied comforts it brings. The Arabs in Tangier drink hot sweet mint tea from tall glasses to cool their bodies on the hottest days. French women drink little cups of it as a tonic, in England it is considered an aphrodisiac, and in the United States it has long been approved as a remedy for flatulence, headache, and nervous tension.

Many women concerned about their skin condition will substitute a mint drink for coffee or regular tea, saying it helps avoid the accumulation of wrinkles brought on by caffein-constricted blood vessels.

VERBENA

The lovely verbena plant with its pale purple flowers and scented leaves offers a delicate lemonlike fragrance to the taste and a soothing brew for an upset stomach. Many times you will notice there is a blotch or blemish on the skin after some stomach distress. This can be the result of the body trying almost immediately to rid itself of toxins and disturbances.

Try a cup of warm verbena tea with a teaspoon of honey after the next upset, and see whether the distress doesn't disappear and the blotch never does appear.

Spanish women know and love verbena tea, and they even have annual fairs—or verbenas, as they call them—stemming from the days when one strolled beyond the city gates to gather masses of the fragrant flowers growing wild on the plains around Madrid.

In France, verbena tea is administered to relieve nervous exhaustion. In addition, lemon verbena leaves brewed into a tea can be taken before bedtime for their soporific effect.

Hippocrates found verbena to be a cure-all, and strongly urged the use of its tea for various indispositions, especially for nervous disorders. This lovely plant has found favor in all civilizations and cultures. Even the Druids probably worshipped the lilac-blossomed plant and chanted gratitude to it for easing their own nervous disorders, stemming from all-night dances in and about Stonehenge.

ELDERFLOWER

Elderflower abounds with testimonials to its effectiveness as a cosmetic or tea. Beautiful women for centuries have jealously guarded their supply of these fragrant flowers. Improvement of skin texture is attributed to a combined cosmetic and tea routine of the blossoms.

According to both old and new herbal sources, elderflower tea, with its rich supply of vitamin P, can help prevent broken veins that mar facial beauty. As a lotion the cold tea is without comparison in its strengthening and gently cleansing and softening action. Taken in frequent enough tisanes, or teas, its action can be mildly laxative, and cleansing to the inner system, too.

Vitamin P, the bioflavonoids, consists of hesperidin, rutin, and citrin and is found mostly in the pulpy portions of fruits and vegetables. By helping to prevent the destruction of vitamin C within the body, vitamin P sources strengthen the fragile capillary walls which, when weakened, break and create the network of red that is so difficult to conceal, even under makeup.

Hippocrates knew the medicinal worth of the elder blossom, plus the plant's bark and root value, and prescribed it for various ailments. Used both internally and externally, it has been considered a cure for eczema. The soothing qualities of this tea make it helpful when you have a headache and, taken before bedtime, it has a tendency to bring sleep more quickly.

CHAMOMILE

And who hasn't heard of the near miracles attributed to the chamomile plant? Tisanes of chamomile are still freely given in European households today as tranquilizers. The pale golden blossom heads are dropped into a cup of boiling water and the tea, sweetened with honey, is taken by those suffering from insomnia or general nervousness.

The feathery flower, smelling of sweet apples, is also taken as a tonic for poor body tone. Because it can revive a tired body and dispirited mind, chamomile tea is sought by those working under pressure for its relaxing qualities. Those who have used this golden herb insist no drug is able to compete with the effectiveness of the chamomile for soothing a harried disposition and restoring calm to a distressed temperament.

ROSE HIPS

Do you want your cheeks to be softly tinted with color? Your eyes to sparkle, and your skin to be supple and well-toned? Rose hips tea can bring a bloom to the wan complexion and better skin texture to the body, if it is vitamin C that is lacking. This ascorbic tea can be considered an excellent tonic because of its high vitamin C content, and in addition it wards off colds, strengthens the gums, and improves the vision. This impressive fruit also hastens the healing process of the entire body.

RASPBERRY

A curiously cooling drink, raspberry tea refreshes even when served warm on a summer's day. Tea made from raspberry leaves was once used to clean the teeth and remove deposits of calculus, or tartar. It is also considered excellent for strengthening the gum tissue around the teeth.

Long used to relieve cramps, raspberry tea has, in addition, become a valued concoction for easing childbirth if taken frequently enough beforehand.

With its valuable vitamin C and iron content, raspberry tea goes high on the beauty list, since many women have iron deficiencies, and this is a pleasant way to supplement your intake of this mineral.

HONEYDEW-MINT LOTION

Give the face a refreshing feast, as melons and mint become available this month. On warm summer days when the face becomes shiny and feels uncomfortably warm, there is nothing more agreeable than a honeydew-mint application. Pat this cooling, cleansing, and tightening astringent lotion into both face and neck and forget about it for an hour. Later, rinse away the lotion in cool water, without using soap, and blot the skin dry.

Recipe for Honeydew-Mint Lotion

Put 2 tablespoons of ripe honeydew melon with 6 to 8 leaves of peppermint into the blender. Start on slow speed and work up to the highest. By now you should have a creamy green lotion of good spreading consistency. Strain through a piece of gauze and bottle for use. Keep refrigerated, but prepare a fresh lotion every 2 days.

Honeydew offers a good source of vitamin C for both diet and cosmetic use, but to vary the formula, substitute cantaloupe or other melon. Cantaloupe will add vitamins A, B, and G (also called B_2), in addition to vitamin C, to your lotion. Use on both face and throat.

FLOWER BEAUTY BATH FOR JUNE

Perfume your personal world by slipping into a tub of crushed, dried flower-petal scents and allowing the delicate odors to bathe your body and send you forth with a perfume as fragile as a nasturtium petal or as mysterious as a wisteria blossom.

June is a month of flowers, so allow your imagination to run wild on selections for a beauty bath. Gather roses, carnations, jasmine, and phlox, lily of the valley, and honeysuckle. Dry the blossoms, fill a bath bag, and suspend it beneath the water faucet in your tub. Let the force of the hot water disperse the exquisite scents and run them into your waiting bath.

Use one or a variety of flowers. Search for the more strongly scented June flowers, the ones that will retain their perfume after being dried. Dry your flower petals first, though. And it is best to prepare a quantity of them and keep them in a covered container, waiting for use. Then, when ready for your bath, dip into the jar and place a cup of blossoms in a gauze bag.

Ninon de L'Enclos' beauty bath was much copied once it became known. This courtesan and beauty of the French court permitted her admirers to believe her favorite bath had much to do with her exquisitely long-lasting beauty. So long did it last, whether from the flower and herb bath or not, that her own grandson inadvertently fell in love with her, having never before met the sparkling lady, when she was seventy years old.

So if you want to try for her brand of fame, drop a handful each of dried rosemary, mint, lavender flowers, and comfrey roots into boiling water, steep, and pour the liquid into your tub. Then place the flower and herbs in a gauze bag and toss it in, too.

Or if you would prefer to use a different mixture, try dried rose geranium leaves, nasturtium, petunias, heliotrope, and lilac together, or singly, by crushing a cupful of the petals and following the above procedure.

STRAWBERRY FACIAL

The rich vitamin C content of ripe strawberries adds to the value of this fruit as a skin tonic. Dull, flaking skin tissue can be rejuvenated and blood circulation stepped up by applications of freshly ripened and crushed berries, if applied frequently enough. Their iron content, when eaten, increases the blood strength and brings color from within.

It is wise to use fresh strawberries both in the diet and as a cosmetic for doubled benefits. A strawberries and cream complexion is not only possible but probable when this routine is added to other good health practices. In earlier times when commercial products were indeed scarce, knowledgeable women gathered dewy fresh berries and mixed them with cream and herbs, or used them plain as a skin rejuvenator.

The practice has never died, and all the smart spas around the world list some form of strawberry in beauty treatments. And now shop counters, too, overflow with pots of cream listed as strawberry mask, lotion, or some other variety of cosmetic. Very few of these contain anything of the original juicy berry. So to be sure you are getting real value, make your own strawberry facial and have the essence.

Strawberry Facial

Place ½ cup of beauty cream base (see page 225) in the blender and beat 1 egg yolk into it. Add ⅓ cup of crushed, fresh, and fully ripe strawberries. Beat until thoroughly blended. Store in a lidded jar in the refrigerator. For hygienic reasons, remove each day the amount you will use as a facial, rather than dipping into it to apply. Rub into the skin in upward, circular motions.

Leave on the skin for a minimum of 30 minutes before washing away in warm and then cool water. Do not use soap in removing the facial. If you think your skin is too oily afterward, mix a few drops of witch hazel in warm water and splash over the face before blotting dry.

MINTED CREAM

Nothing produces so pungently the sensation of freshness and life as summer mint, picked from the vine. This herb is even crisp in scent, and when you use it as a cosmetic or add it to a skin preparation, you can feel the immediate tingly results of increased stimulation from this trusty beauty plant. Take every opportunity to use fresh mint in your cosmetic preparations. If you cannot get the fresh plant, then resort to the dried leaf and restore it to life with a splash of hot water over the leaves, allowing them to steep before draining off the mint water, and use it just like the fresh.

Try the minted face cream listed here, and feel the summer's freshness that is added to this rather standard cosmetic mixture.

Minted Face Cream

5 ounces lanolin	4 ounces mineral water
3 ounces sweet almond oil	1 ounce strong mint tea

Melt the lanolin over hot water and beat in the almond oil, water, and mint tea. Beat until fluffy and pour into a cosmetic jar with a lid. Use as a covering for dry or normal skin

YARROW HAIR RINSE

Herbs contribute a lasting and beneficially strengthening effect to both skin and scalp. They are cleansing and stimulating, according to the plant used, and you can select the quality you require from a vast array in a herbalist's shop, a botanical supply house, or a health food company featuring dried herbs. Better yet, if you've space, you can grow your own. Or you can learn to identify them and gather many of them along roadsides, in pastures, and in the woods.

Rich in copper, yarrow is one of the finest herbs, and it can be found growing wild almost anywhere, it is so prolific. A brew of yarrow plant made into a lotion is supposed to stop falling hair. Its tonic properties dilate the pore openings and rush its benefits to a distressed scalp.

If you are using freshly pulled yarrow leaves, drop a good handful into 2 cups of boiling water. Steep until lukewarm and massage the liquid into the hair after a shampoo as the final rinse.

If you have purchased dried yarrow, use 1 ounce for every 2 cups of boiling water and proceed as with the fresh leaves.

ELDERFLOWER WATER

Making some natural beauty preparations is as simple as turning to the kitchen pantry, and refrigerator, and garden and whipping them up; others, however, require a little research and patience. But the rewards are great and the results cannot be achieved by any other method, so it really resolves itself to a question of how much you value a lovely appearance.

Preparing elderflower water falls into this category. It is not complicated to prepare the water, but you must know your botany well enough to recognize an elderflower tree or be willing to purchase the dried flowers and beat up the potion yourself, for it simply does not exist in prepared form on the market today. Although the distilled type is far better, you can nevertheless prepare the water by the easy boiling method in small enough quantities to prevent spoilage and thus have a similar preparation.

When picking the flowers, cut them off the stalks near the blossoms. Place the flowers in an enameled saucepan. Cover with water and bring to a boiling point, then pour through a gauze to strain out the blossoms. Bottle for use and keep refrigerated.

Another way to use the softening qualities and perfume of the elderflower is to pack an earthenware jar full of the blossoms. Pour hot, but not boiling, water over the contents, cover, and leave for twenty-four hours. Strain this liquid through a double layer of gauze or muslin to remove all particles. This, too, should be refrigerated, but half an ounce of simple tincture of benzoin or two ounces of alcohol will help preserve it.

Elderflower water has been a favorite complexion wash for centuries. It endured at least from medieval days until well into this century, when it was ousted by commercial creams, soaps, and lotions—none of which can give the softening effects of this scented flower lotion.

So use it as a refreshing face wash, alone, without soap, by dipping a cotton ball into the liquid and gently patting it into the face with upward circular motions.

Until you find out how much of this fragrant liquid you will be using, it would probably be best to try the first method, remembering at the same time that you can always share these homemade beauty preparations with a friend.

ASTRINGENT LOTION FOR ENLARGED PORES

Now that you have made your plain elderflower water, you can use it with the juice of a cucumber to produce a refreshing lotion to help contract large pores and refine the skin. An old formula suggests you take a half-pint bottle and place in it the juice of 1 cucumber, or about 2 or 3 tablespoons. Fill the bottle half full with elderflower water and shake well to blend the two liquids. Very slowly add ½ ounce of simple tincture of benzoin and shake again. Fill the remainder of the bottle with elderflower water and shake well before capping it.

This is supposed to keep well without refrigeration, but since this is a rather large quantity, it might be wise to keep one half of it refrigerated (or cut the amount in half). But be sure to label this lotion, and all others, that you place in the refrigerator to prevent its being used as a food.

Use on a clean skin daily to help close pores and firm the skin.

APHRODISIAC FOR JUNE

Orange blossoms have been associated with love for all the centuries since crusading knights returned with the chaste flower and exotic fruit as their victor's spoils. Later, a bouquet of orange blossoms was usually a gift from a man to the woman he loved just before he married her.

So traditional is the custom of orange blossoms at weddings that the delicate blossoms immediately summon thoughts of soft music, beauty, and restrained passion. To step up the tempo a bit, and because orange blossoms aren't all that accessible, let's try an orange puree that excites the mind and taste buds.

Besides, what's wrong with starting a relationship with oranges instead of wasting all that time being traditional? That part is fine, but there's no reason to stint on anything that brings the end closer to the beginning.

Heat 2 cups of fresh orange juice in a saucepan. Beat in 1 teaspoon of arrowroot mixed with 2 tablespoons of cold water. Cook until clear and stir in ½ cup orange blossom honey with 2 teaspoons of grated orange rind. Chill and serve as a dessert.

LEG EXERCISES

Legs that seemed in good shape in jeans, heavy slacks, or pantsuits all winter now sometimes emerge as less than perfect. June is bikini time, but even if you prefer a body suit, your thighs are still going to show.

It seems unfair that men seldom have bulging thighs while the majority of American women are afflicted with this problem. And with life becoming more and more sedentary for so many, this area of the body will spread even more rapidly, at even earlier ages.

Pile into your exercises and trim the excess flesh away from your thighs before summer comes any closer. Re-create a compact, feminine line which doesn't shout of childbirth, housekeeping, and Mother Hubbard concealers. You can regain a sylphlike thigh line if you dedicate yourself to the following exercises with a determination to be as trim as you once were.

Sit on the floor with your legs extended before you. Slowly draw your legs up until your heels are as near your body as possible. Now, open your knees and allow them to lean to either side. Place the soles of your feet together and, holding the toes with your hands, have the knees touch the floor or come as close to the floor as is comfortably possible.

Do not force the knees down. Daily practice will cause them gradually to lower as the hip tendons and thigh muscles stretch and become more elastic. Straighten the legs and return them to their prone position. Repeat several times.

Lie on your right side and support your head on your hand, with the elbow against the floor. Very slowly raise the left leg ceilingward as high as possible and hold it there for a moment. Slowly bring it down, turn over to the left side, and repeat. This should pull on the inner thighs for toning and control.

Lying on your back, very slowly raise your buttocks in the air, aiding the ascent by "walking" your hands up the spine toward the middle of the back for support. Use both hands to support the back as high up as possible. Now, slowly spread the legs to either side, as far as they will reach, making a Y shape. Hold them at that angle for a moment and bring them back again before swinging them out once more. Repeat several times, or as long as this is comfortable.

Extra weight simply cannot be removed from the thigh area by diet alone. In fact, when weight loss occurs without proper exercise, there is a tendency toward flabbiness and skin-tone loss. This area of the body requires daily flexing in order to regain control when the thighs begin to spread in unattractive flesh gain.

While some health and beauty clubs have various rollers and beater-type equipment which are supposed to break down excess fat on the thighs and tone the general area, this equipment can be harmful by breaking, instead, the surface blood vessels where they pound or roll or beat. This area should remain strictly a do-it-yourself project, without the use of extra equipment.

BREAKFASTS FOR JUNE

Strawberries, honey, and milk
Poached eggs with chives
Whole grain bread
Herbal tea

Blueberries and honey
Brown rice with raisins
Herbal tea

Pineapple and strawberry cup
Oatcakes (recipe on p. 69) with honey and nut butter
Herbal tea

Strawberry soya shake*
Scrambled eggs with mung sprouts
Sesame seed toast with honey
Herbal tea

Fresh cherries
Granola (recipe on p. 21)
Herbal tea

Mixed fresh fruit
Brown rice flour pancakes with strawberry sauce (recipe on p. 21)
Herbal tea

Strawberry soya shake*
Omelette Lyonnaise
Herbal tea

LUNCHES FOR JUNE

❧

Asparagus soup*
Watercress, hard-boiled-egg sandwiches
Yogurt

Cauliflower soup (recipe on p. 118)
Chef salad with soya sprouts
Yogurt

Spring salad of greens—dandelion, violet, and lettuce
Eggs with yogurt and chives*
Yogurt

Avocado soup*
Radish, carrot, and beet salad
Yogurt

Green pea soup (recipe on p. 118)
Young beet-top salad
Almond butter (recipe on p. 202) whole wheat sandwiches
Yogurt

Cherries, cottage cheese, and almond salad
Nasturtium whole wheat sandwiches*
Yogurt

DINNERS FOR JUNE

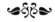

Broiled liver
Carrots and mint
Steamed dandelion greens

Seed nut patties*
Baked potatoes
Chard, dandelion, or other greens

Fresh salmon
Marigold-rice pilaf*
Asparagus

Lentil loaf (recipe on p. 22)
Carrots
Peas

Kidney with broiled tomatoes
Summer squash
Green beans

Cheese soufflé
Fresh lima beans
Tomatoes

Sautéed brains
Asparagus
Beets

RECIPES FOR JUNE

Strawberry Soya Shake

2 cups cold water	honey to taste
½ cup fresh strawberries	2 tablespoons soya powder
½ cup fresh pineapple	

Liquefy in blender.

Asparagus Soup

Blend together 1 cup chopped cooked asparagus, 2 cups of milk, and a pinch of mace. Use hot or cold milk, according to preference, and heated or cold asparagus. Adjust the amount of milk used for thinner or thicker consistency.

Eggs with Yogurt and Chives

4 eggs	2 tablespoons sweet butter
4 slices whole grain bread	minced chives
1 cup yogurt	seasoning

Cut the largest round possible from bread slice. From that, cut out a circle large enough to hold an egg. Toast the rings and butter them. Place on a baking sheet and drop a raw egg into the center of each ring of bread. Sprinkle with seasoning and cover each yolk with yogurt and chives. Bake at 350 degrees until the eggs are set.

Avocado Soup

Peel and quarter one avocado. Place with 2 cups milk, 1 cup chicken broth, and 1 leaf of basil into the blender and beat smooth. Pour into saucepan and heat slowly.

Nasturtium Whole Wheat Sandwiches

Mince a handful of nasturtium leaves and mix into a tablespoon or more of sweet butter. Spread on whole grain bread.

Seed Nut Patties

1 cup pecan meal	½ cup grated potato
½ cup whole grain cracker meal	1 cup milk
2 tablespoons minced onion	1 tablespoon vegetable or nut oil
2 tablespoons minced celery	seasoning
¾ cup sunflower meal	

Mix all ingredients together and bake in oiled loaf pan for one hour at 350 degrees. Serve with sauce.

Marigold-Rice Pilaf

1 cup brown rice	3 cups chicken broth
5 tablespoons vegetable oil	seasoning
½ cup marigold petals	

Heat the rice in the oil in a heavy skillet until it appears to be browning. Sprinkle the petals over the rice and pour in the chicken broth. Cover and cook until tender. Stir in salt or other seasoning.

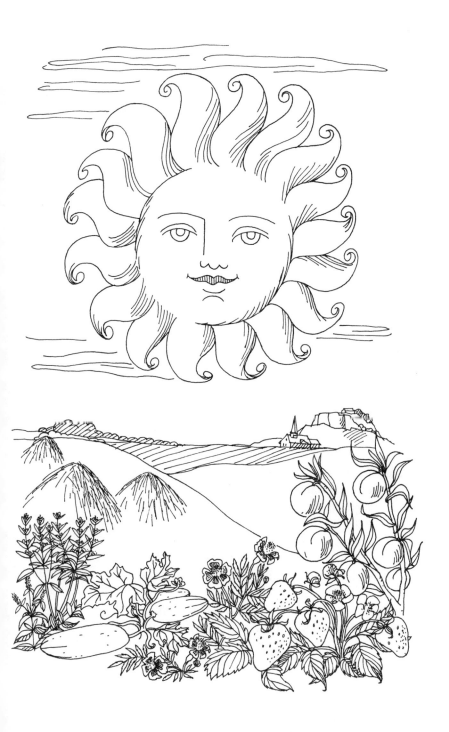

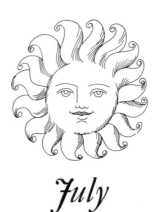

July

I remember, I remember,
How my childhood fleeted by,
The mirth of its December,
And the warmth of its July.

> *Winthrop Praed: "I Remember"*

Mark Anthony named this month in honor of Julius Caesar. It was later called Hay Month and Harvest Month on the French calendar. And it is the time for frolicking through warm days, of courting the sunshine cautiously but pleasurably, of taking all the produce of the land that will add to comfort and beauty. There are cucumbers in all their brilliance waiting to refresh the skin in a chill and soothing lotion, peaches and cream to be eaten and worn like a blush upon the cheeks. Flowers bloom to be petaled on a salad and herbs to be made into a rinse for dull hair. This is indeed the fruitful season for those summer things that come quickly and disappear before the harvest of sturdier staples.

So wake up your sleeping body and let it know its complete power when allied with nature. Try an air bath for refreshment, softening its assault from the sun by lathering in a suntan lotion and, should you overdo it, removing the sting of overexposure with a comforting barley paste. Be like a bronze-haired Aztec princess and pour the shine of marigold brew upon your hair— and realize that July will not last for long, as no perfect thing seems to.

AIR BATHS

For all the years of our lives we are covered with layers of clothing. Except for brief moments, the skin on our bodies seldom has a chance to breathe without obstruction. An air bath is a delightful and rewarding respite from all the hours of swaddling confinement we undergo.

Exposing the body to air is an ancient custom, practiced by those who have found a sense of refreshment in leaving the body unclothed for a period of time each day. This is, of course, more easily practiced in warmer climates, but even in colder areas you can use the spring, summer, and fall to advantage.

Probably more people than you realize have discovered this luxurious practice that takes no additional time and gives the body freshness and invigoration. Benjamin Franklin, always modern in his outlook and frankly curious about getting the most out of living, practiced air bathing with much pleasure. Every morning at daybreak it was his custom to arise and spend about an hour writing or reading in his room without any clothes on.

The effect of air and sunlight directly on the skin is most agreeable. With today's scant bathing suits the young can experience this benefit more fully than those who wear more modest bathing suits. But few people swim daily, and for an air bath to be entirely effective, the body should be completely uncovered. Perhaps Franklin's early morning hour is not for you, for he did live alone, off and on. If not his hour, then choose a more convenient time.

Find a private place in your home. Of course, a terrace screened from view would be ideal, but it is not sun we want as much as air. Even an open window will serve admirably. You might even like to use your slantboard during this time, to combine the two periods and get more mileage out of limited time.

There is something absolutely delicious about air bathing, or permitting the body pores to breathe without restriction every day. The results are similar to an invigorating exercise or a stimulating tub bath.

Probably after you experience the pleasurable air bath, you will become more tolerant or understanding about nudist colonies and their insistence on bareness as a means of bodily comfort and health. But if you are of a conservative bent yet still want all that is best for your body, air bathing can be strictly a private experience, practiced without anyone's being the wiser.

An easy, practical way to air bathe is by simply sleeping without restricting pajamas or gowns. Usually this is merely habit, anyway, and since there is bed clothing surrounding you, what need have you of additional covering? Deeper and more tranquil slumber will usually result from sleeping nude. And sleep seems to come more quickly when you are unhampered by clothing in bed. So throw your window open wide, retire for the night, and allow your pores to be refreshed and renewed by additional oxygen intake.

SUNTAN LOTIONS

The damage done to the skin during the summer months from overindulgence in the sun is inestimable. Moderate amounts of all of nature are desirable and rewarding, but constant or too frequent dalliance with summer sun, when the rays are more direct, can destroy body tissue to such a point that a person can age several years in appearance in a few short months.

Treat the sun as a friend, but do not embrace it on a daily basis. If you do, not only are you damaging the skin you ordinarily pamper, but you are also courting disaster in the form of skin cancer, coming from overexposure. Too many women now in their forties are paying for the overenthusiastic sunbathing that became a favorite pastime when they were in their teens and twenties.

Dry, leathery skin results from too much tanning. In fact, sometimes a tanned animal hide appears to have as much life as the complexion of those women who have overexposed themselves to the sun's ultraviolet rays.

If you insist upon sunbathing to acquire a tan, there are some applications which will promote it and so get you out of the sun that much sooner. At the same time, they offer some bit of protection to the skin in helping ward off the dry-cooked appearance that can result from too much sun.

Suntanning Cream

½ cup sesame seed oil
1 egg yolk
1 tablespoon wheat germ oil

1 tablespoon lemon juice
mint leaves

Blend together all the ingredients, except the mint leaves, in the blender until thick. Add 1 teaspoon of mint juice crushed from the leaves, or made by beating 1 or 2 tablespoons of water with a handful of mint leaves in the blender before beginning. Rub into the body before exposing it to the sun. Keep refrigerated when not in use.

Another excellent suntan lotion can be made by grinding a handful of sesame seeds in a grinder to produce a powder. Add enough water to form a milky fluid, strain, and apply the liquid to all areas of the body that will be exposed to the sun. Reapply each time after entering the water. This soft and velvety lotion will produce a beautifully even tan.

FOOT EASE IN JULY

This month, for all its pleasures, brings with it foot care problems you usually don't have during the colder months. Tired, aching, and burning feet can stem from too much walking in poorly fitting shoes which do not allow enough ventilation for the feet. Apple cider vinegar is an old and effective means of comforting aching feet. First wash the feet well in warm water, then plunge them into cool water or hold them beneath the tub faucet after a warm foot bath and allow a stimulating current of cool water to play over them for several minutes. Dry thoroughly and rub a tablespoon of vinegar into the sole of each foot. Continue to massage lightly until the foot is completely dry.

When perspiration becomes disagreeable, a foot bath laced with spirits of camphor can be pleasantly effective. Use a tablespoon of spirits of camphor to a basin of water.

CUCUMBER FRESHENER

Summer sun and heat seem to produce more oily areas on the face than are seen at any other time of the year. Instead of washing the face frequently and removing its protective acid mantle, try a refreshing and nourishing cucumber skin freshener which will rinse away the patches of oil, but leave the complexion fresh and supple.

Cucumber Freshener

Drop half a scrubbed and chopped cucumber into the blender. Be sure it is not waxed. If it is oiled, remove the oil by scrubbing with warm water and apple cider vinegar and drying it well. If it still appears oily, peel the skin and use only the inside of the cucumber.

After reducing the cucumber to a pulp in the blender, squeeze it through gauze to extract all the juice. Add 1 teaspoon of witch hazel to ½ cup of cucumber juice. Chill and use with cotton balls to cleanse the skin of oil during the day. Keep refrigerated.

BARLEY PASTE FOR SUNBURN

When overenthusiasm for a tan has made you incautious and the results are an uncomfortable sunburn, an old-fashioned barley paste can be very soothing and help to reduce the redness.

Grind three ounces of unpearled barley, and mix the powder with one ounce of raw honey. Blend into a smooth paste and add the unbeaten white of one egg. The final result should be a smooth paste. Gently rub this into the affected area and allow to remain on overnight if possible, or most of the day, for the best results. Remember, the old-fashioned methods of beauty care are longer lasting than modern cosmetics or medications, which can have uncomfortable side effects. At the same time, the home-prepared remedies and treatments require longer to be effective. Nature will do its work perfectly, but it won't be rushed.

A SWEET BAG FOR SCENTING

For a pleasant summer's day occupation, make a Sweet Bag for tucking away in linen drawers and closets. July brings roses in quantity for those who have nourished their bushes, especially for those who have reinstated the old-fashioned Damask rose in their gardens. For them the job is easy and the results are delightful.

Dry 4 quarts of fresh rose petals in an airy place. Stir them daily to ensure proper drying; if you dry them outdoors, bring them in each night to avoid dampness. When they are dry and softly scented, proceed with the following items:

8 ounces grated dried orange peel	½ ounce crushed sweet marjoram leaves
8 ounces grated dried lemon peel	8 ounces powdered Sweet Flag
8 ounces powdered orris root	½ ounce powdered cloves
½ ounce powdered nutmeg	⅛ teaspoon musk
2 ounces ground coriander seeds	⅛ teaspoon ambergris
	1 teaspoon rose oil

Use your mortar and pestle, blender, or grinder, to produce a powder of the lemon and orange peel. Mix ingredients together, sprinkle with 1 teaspoon of rose oil, and tuck into little cotton bags to place among your linens or wherever you want an exquisite scent.

PEACHES AND CREAM SKIN SOFTENER

There is something absolutely beautiful about a bowl of fresh peaches and real cream. The fruit looks sun-kissed and warm and alive with color, and the ivory richness of the cream crowns the fruit. Why not wear it and eat it, too? This nutritious and beautiful dessert will then do twice as much for you. Fresh peaches offer you a feast of vitamins A, B, and C, along with calcium for serenity and magnesium for good skin. Add to that vitamin D from certified fresh, raw cream for lagniappe, or a little something extra, as the New Orleans French Creoles say.

Mash to a pulp a tablespoon of a completely ripe peach. Mix in enough cream to make a thick application. Lie down on your slantboard and apply a generous layer of the fruit and cream to your face and neck. Allow the mixture to remain on the face for thirty minutes. Remove and rinse the face in warm and then cool water several times. Gently pat away the excess moisture without rubbing. Do not use soap.

And since this is an edible cosmetic, get double duty by doubling the quantity, your weight permitting, adding a dollop of honey, and eating it after your facial. You'll tingle outside and in.

NETTLE HAIR RINSE

Fortify the hair for its dose of summer sun, seawater, and chlorinated pool water by shampooing weekly with strengthening herbs. Hair that is in good condition, with strong roots and sturdy strands, will be more resistant to the summer's assaults on it.

Nettle wash is a prized formula for promoting tissue strength and improving hair texture. Its use has brought praise for its virtues down through the centuries. In addition to other qualities, it also is an excellent wash for removing dandruff, and at the same time it improves the color of the hair.

Early herbalists invariably prescribed a daily dip into nettle lotion and a combing through the hair to lend body. If you gather the leaves yourself, be sure to wear gloves and to use shears for snipping, for the formic acid found in the fresh green leaves creates blisters on contact with the skin. After gathering the nettle leaves, allow them to dry before crumbling and using them as a rinse. It is easier, and perhaps wiser, to purchase the nettle leaves from a health food store, herbalist, or botanical supply house. They are safe to handle in a dry state.

Add to the nettle crumbled leaves of sage, which also stimulates hair growth and in this way increases the benefit of the herbal rinse.

Mix together ½ cup each of nettle and sage and cover for later use. Pour 2 cups of boiling water over ¼ cup of the combined mixture for each rinse, allowing it to steep until warm to the touch. Strain and use after shampooing and rinsing the hair thoroughly. Place a small basin beneath the head and pour the nettle-sage rinse over the hair several times. Then massage the hair for several minutes and pour one last rinse over it. Wrap a towel around the head for 5 minutes or so before setting, or further preparing the hair.

LIQUID DEODORANT FOR THE SUMMER

Summertime is upon us and the desire to exercise more by participating in outdoor activities in homage to the season brings with it a problem. We know that many commerical deodorants contain an aluminum compound or other harmful ingredient, and consequently we are uncertain what to do to avoid body odor.

According to an observer of the nineteenth century, perspiration is nature's effort to cleanse the skin, and baths are man's attempt to do the same thing.

But more than a bath is needed in the summertime to remain free of offensive odors which come, not from perspiration, but from bacteria acting upon the moisture exuded from the skin.

Until you can find a harmless and effective deodorant with no deleterious chemicals which may produce their own ills, perhaps you would like to make your own. An old-fashioned and respected formula is beautiful in its simplicity. According to the instructions, boil a few ounces of oak bark (available from a botanical supply house) for 15 minutes in a quart of water. Strain and bottle the liquid and mix a couple tablespoons of it to ½ cup of water for bathing the underarms.

For excessive perspiration, you might want to try another old practice from the days before roll-ons and sprays.

In 1 quart of boiling water mix together ½ ounce of powdered alum with ¼ ounce of powdered camphor and the juice and peel of 1 lemon. Dissolve by stirring and bottle for use. After bathing, apply the liquid to the underarm area and allow to dry.

Another simple method of removing perspiration odors from the body is to gather one or two chrysanthemum leaves and crush them until they are soft and moist. Rub them gently under the arms and you will find you have a most effective deodorizer without stopping the flow of perspiration, which is a natural and beneficial action of the body.

Powdered starch placed in a flannel bag and wet thoroughly with bay rum has proved a refreshing and cooling toilet powder for those affected by excessive perspiration who develop heat rashes from their own perspiration.

FRECKLES

At one time, when freckles weren't as casually accepted as today, women fought them off with various concoctions they brewed or had made up. They also gave them names to lessen their supposed blight. Sun kisses and the kisses of Apollo were two favorite expressions meant to take the sting from the freckled face. Beauty books soothed heavily freckled young girls by telling them a few freckles under the eyes increased their beauty by enhancing their expression and calling attention to their eyes—or that Cleopatra was "with Phoebus's amorous pinches black." Over the years, more charming than accurate explanations have been given of the little rusty wonders that will allow themselves to be bleached a bit, covered somewhat, but disposed of never.

One nineteenth-century explanation suggested freckles consist of iron in the blood combining with the light of day. The minute iron portions supposedly found themselves outside the usual tract of skin and deposited themselves just under the surface of top skin. When exposed to light, the particles immediately turned darker and thus freckles were born.

Today, dermatologists aren't overly concerned about freckles, so matter of factly are they accepted. And their explanation is that they are small accumulations of pigment which have not been evenly distributed throughout the skin. Sunlight does in fact, tend to darken them, so avoiding heavy doses of sun will help prevent the deepening color that seems to distress those overly burdened with this pigmented spotting.

Fading freckles are about the most one can hope for. There seem to be two types. "Cold," or winter, freckles, as they have been known for some time, are the more permanent type. Summer freckles appear only in that season and intensify or diminish according to exposure to the sun. They tend to disappear in winter. Winter freckles come to stay. Lotions and bleaches will help soften the color of both summer and winter freckles. If the freckles really distress you, they can be "painted" with a camel's hair brush dipped into lemon juice every night; the dried juice should be allowed to remain until morning. Rinse the face and apply a thin coating of salad oil. If the skin shows signs of irritation, add plain water or rose water to the lemon juice to weaken it. Discontinue the use altogether if it becomes uncomfortable.

Buttermilk or yogurt are two excellent skin bleaches but, as with the lemon juice, they must be applied daily in order to be effective.

STRAWBERRY PASTE
TO REFRESH THE SKIN

In July, pour all of summertime's wealth into your body. Too soon the fruits of summer will be gone, and you will be left with tasteless foods which have lost much of their vitamin and mineral value because they have been shipped enormous distances.

Pick a basket, or pick up a basket, of little, red, ripe strawberries to eat and to use as a cosmetic. In this manner you can grow strawberries in your own cheeks. Make strawberry lotions and custards and paste, and prepare bowls of strawberries and honey and milk. Use the berries in every conceivable way, and if you are in a hurry, just bite the end from one and rub the rich red juice onto an oily skin or a skin that needs moisture, bleaching, cleansing, or reviving. Rinse away after it has dried and note the color in your complexion.

Strawberry Paste to Refresh the Complexion

⅙ ounce gum tragacanth
rose water, orange water, or
elderflower water

½ pound fresh, ripe straw-
berries

Soak the gum tragacanth in enough rose water to soften to a thin mucilage. Chop and crush the strawberries. They *must* be ripe for this formula; no half-ripe or too-firm berry will do. Mix the berries with rose water to form a liquid paste. Beat in the tragacanth. Store in a capped jar in the refrigerator when not in use.

Gently massage the paste into the face and neck area at night, in order to soften and tone the skin. Rinse away with warm water in the morning.(You might want to protect the bedding by using an old pillowcase.)

Strawberries, along with citrus fruits and some vegetables, are an important source of bioflavonoids, which are used effectively in treating skin hemorrhage among other ailments. This condition is caused when blood vessel walls are so fragile they erupt and leave spidery red lines across a face. Since this is a frequent cosmetic misery, it would be very wise to add these luscious fruits to the diet during their season, and when their all-too-brief appearance is over, substituting other sources of the important bioflavonoid.

THROAT LIGHTENER

Midsummer, and is your neck still a dream, or has it become mottled and spotted with sun and salt wind exposure? When attempting to get a tan, some women find the neck area offers resistance to an evenness of color. After a vacation at the shore, or even after the relatively small exposure of just walking around the shopping center, this sensitive part of the body can develop problems which won't go away without your assistance.

The yellow/red/brown neck mosaic that can shriek unkind things about your age must be toned down, removed, or covered. No makeup can perform the job adequately. However, the following cosmetic bleach will usually restore evenness of color, degrees lighter than its present state, while softening and toning because of the valuable nutrients.

Blend 1 ounce of honey with 1 teaspoonful of lemon juice. Beat in 6 drops of oil of bitter almonds, and stir in 2 egg whites. Whirl oatmeal in a blender or nut grinder until it is a powder, and then add enough to the liquid to make a smooth paste.

Apply to the discolored neck area and allow to remain overnight or several hours during the day. Remove with warm water and add a thin film of sesame or other seed, nut, or vegetable oil. Keep remainder in the refrigerator and remove just enough to warm to room temperature before applying to the skin.

APHRODISIAC FOR JULY

There has to be a rose aphrodisiac which will stun the senses and tune in the soul. Honey of Roses is one such treat. Just thinking of deep-scented rose petals brings on warmth and pleasure. In earlier times, roses were fed to lovers in an unending succession of passionate dishes such as Damask Rose Syrup, Conserve of Roses, Rose Wafers, and Eglantine Sauce.

Beds were strewn with rose petals in Grecian ceremonies, and petals were tossed out upon Roman orgies even as jets of rose water were sprayed over the participants. If you can find an unsprayed source of roses, the following recipe sounds promising. It has all the minerals that honey provides, it tastes good, and its scent is pleasing, too.

4 ounces unsprayed rose petals   2 pounds honey (clover or
2 cups boiling water   other light variety)

Put the roses in a stone, enamel, or glass container and pour the
boiling water over them. Steep overnight and strain the liquid
from the petals by pressing them against a sieve to extract all the
flavor and color. Add the liquid to a 2-pound jar of clover or other
light honey. Simmer to a thick syrup consistency and store for use.

HIP EXERCISES FOR JULY

Bathing suit too tight? Bulging out the edges? That's no way
to face the summer. A season of fireside sitting can play havoc with
a figure and sound the death knell for a pleasurable summer.
Somehow, with our figures hidden away, the picture we carry of
ourselves is usually a great deal more flattering than it actually is.

Strip away the layers of clothing and pull on shorts, a bikini,
or even a simple summer dress, and all the nice secrets of heavier
clothing disappear. You are left with deposits of dimples and
ripples where firm flesh should be. No need to worry. Daily battle
in the form of mild body movement will chase away the most
stubborn roll of flesh. Even around the hips, where women seem
to expand first, enlarging dimensions can be halted and the figure
regained.

Spreading hips suggest middle-aged debilitation, but today a
large number of young girls have this unattractive condition, too.
Sedentary jobs, television watching, aversion to exercise, and little
or no real walking catapult them into this state.

A tried and true hip-swinging exercise and reducer requires
you to lie on the floor flat and comfortably on your back. Extend
your arms to either side at shoulder level to rest on the floor.
Breathing deeply in and out—for one has a tendency to shallow

breathe in this movement and deprive the body of needed oxygen—swing the right leg from the hip over to touch the fingers of the left hand.

It may not be possible to reach this point, but the hand is the ideal goal. Slowly swing the leg back and lower it to the floor. Repeat with the left leg, swinging it over to touch the right fingers. Repeat several times.

Don't miss a single day on this body movement and you will have your hips in sylph form in shorter time than you would have believed possible.

Another exercise that gets at the bulging hip finds you lying on your side on the floor. For comfort's sake, you can support your head on your folded arm, but remain lying on your side. Very slowly glide your foot and leg along the floor toward your arm. According to your physical condition, you will probably get only waist high with your foot. But if your body has been long neglected, you may be able to glide it no higher than a foot or two. Do not force it any higher. Daily practice will limber the hip muscles and at the same time work away excess flesh. Turn on the other side and repeat with the other leg.

Some women are loath to try any but stand-up exercises. They say they don't mind exercising off and on all day as long as they don't have to lie down for the movements. For these people, the following is a quickie that can be done at odd moments during the day.

Stand behind a heavy chair and place both hands on the chair back. Bend the right leg in order to bring the knee in as close as possible toward the chest. Dip your head to meet your knee and then slowly drop the leg and swing it backward to form a straight line behind you. Relax and return the leg to a standing position. Repeat with the left leg. Begin cautiously, performing this movement only two or three times the first day. Gradually work up to half a dozen times.

BREAKFASTS FOR JULY

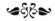

Bowl of strawberries, honey, and milk
Soy pancakes
Herbal tea

Bowl of peaches and milk
Poached eggs fines herbes
Corn muffins
Herbal tea

Honeydew and mint leaves
Granola (recipe on p. 21)
Herbal tea

Mélange of strawberries, blueberries, and peaches
Brown rice and raisins
Herbal tea

Melon with raspberries
Apple pancake*
Herbal tea

Bowl of fresh cherries
Oatmeal soaked overnight with raisins
Herbal tea

Fresh fruit cup
Omelet with fresh honeyed peaches
Wheat toast
Herbal tea

LUNCHES FOR JULY

Cream of broccoli soup with nasturtium buds*
Cheese and tomato sandwiches
Yogurt

Raw salad bowl
Sardine sandwiches
Yogurt

Rice, tomato, pepper, and radish salad
Crackers and cheese
Yogurt

Herb soup*
Chinese cabbage salad
Yogurt

Beet borscht (recipe on p. 93)
Watermelon balls and mint leaves
Yogurt

Shredded carrot, apple, and raisin salad
Wheat germ muffins (recipe on p. 92) and cheese
Yogurt

Corn soup*
Cottage cheese and green salad
Yogurt

DINNERS FOR JULY

Cheese soufflé
Peas and minced lettuce cooked together
Coleslaw

Broiled liver and tomatoes
Parsleyed potatoes
Corn on the cob

Cold salmon
Mushrooms stuffed with rice and herbs
French potato salad

Sweetbreads with fresh chives
Corn pudding
Raw spinach and sweet onion salad

Vegetable casserole*
Corn sticks
Tomatoes stuffed with coleslaw

Broiled fish
Beets
Shredded cabbage salad

Meatless meat loaf*
Asparagus
Corn on the cob

RECIPES FOR JULY

Apple Pancake

3 apples, thinly sliced	2 beaten eggs
⅓ cup vegetable oil	½ cup milk
⅓ cup honey	½ cup whole grain flour
nutmeg	¼ teaspoon sea salt
cinnamon	4 tablespoons vegetable oil

Cook apple slices in oil until just tender. Mix honey and spices and mix into apples and cook 10 minutes longer. Remove from heat and cool. Beat together eggs, flour, milk, and salt. Pour enough of remaining oil into heavy pan to cover sides and bottom and heat. When very hot, pour in the batter and bake in hot oven —450 degrees—for 15 to 20 minutes. Watch for the center of the pancake to rise up and puncture it. Continue baking until it becomes golden brown. Remove from oven and spread the apple mixture over the pancake and fold. Dribble additional honey over the pancake and serve hot.

Cream of Broccoli Soup with Nasturtium Buds

See recipe on page 47 for soup. Sprinkle with fresh flower buds.

Herb Soup

1 tablespoon arrowroot   1 minced shallot
2 cups chicken or fish stock   lemon peel, minced
1 tablespoon salad oil
1 teaspoon each minced
    parsley, sweet basil, chives,
    and tarragon

Stir arrowroot into enough stock to make a thin paste. Heat remaining stock and stir in first mixture. Simmer for 5 minutes. Sauté the herbs and shallot in the oil and add to the thickened soup. Serve with finely minced lemon peel stirred into the hot soup at the last minute.

Corn Soup

Cut 2 cups of raw corn off the cob and add with the following in the blender.

1 cup minced celery   pinch of sea salt
¼ cup minced green pepper   1 cup milk
1 teaspoon vegetable oil

Blend at high speed and heat for 5 minutes in a saucepan. Thin with additional milk if desired.

Vegetable Casserole

Combine 1 cup each of fresh chopped tomatoes, fresh lima beans, fresh corn, 1 minced onion, and 1 cup puréed peas, just mixed, with ½ cup grated natural or Swiss cheese. Sprinkle more cheese on top and bake in oiled casserole in oven at 350 degrees until done.

Meatless Meat Loaf

2 potatoes in skin	2 eggs, beaten
1½ cups pecans	seasoning: 1 teaspoon minced
1 cup onions	basil
1 cup whole wheat crumbs	

Put potatoes, pecans, onions, and crumbs through a food mill and grind fine. Mix in eggs and basil and put in an oiled loaf pan. Bake at 350 degrees until done, about 1 hour.

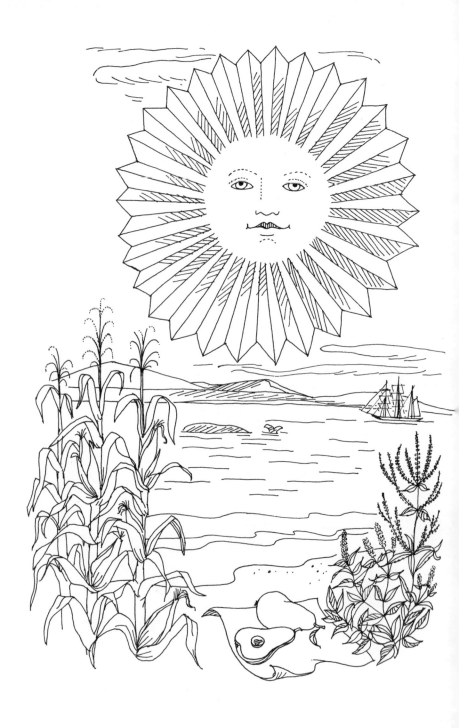

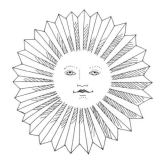

August

*Rejoice! ye fields, rejoice! and wave
with gold,
When August round her precious gifts
is flinging;
Lo! the crushed wain is slowly
homeward rolled:
The sunburnt reapers jocund lays are
singing.*

        John Ruskin: "The Months"

Augustus, the Roman emperor, gave this stately period of time his name and considered it his lucky month, as indeed it is for all in its sumptuous offerings. In earlier centuries, it was called the Weed Month, Harvest Month, and Hot Month, and it probably was all of those.

But August also was the time to look around and accept all that is offered from nature, for this is the last month for the quick-growing things that become fresh, summer foods on which one depends for vitality and attractiveness. There is corn on the stalk, to eat from the cob and to cut from it for a facial feast. Raw corn milk makes the skin satiny, and wise women have always used it as a special complexion milk, knowing its nutritious qualities.

There is mint on the vine, to swirl up into a cooling lotion or to mix with a shampoo for a refreshing change and air-fresh cleanliness. Watermelon can tinge a cheek with color, and help to paint summer's warm glow on your skin. At the same time, look closely at your fingernails and check to see whether your love of the earth and gardening—or your casual attitude—has affected them. Strengthen and pamper them with a lovely rose food.

Reach gratefully for these beauty aids and, like Augustus, consider this your lucky month.

FINGERNAILS

Fingernails, like other parts of the body, quickly reflect inadequate nutrition. Lack of protein or faulty assimilation usually results in poorly formed and slow-growing nails. In this sense, they are an indication of your general health.

In some parts of the world, the appearance of the fingernails is of great importance. Spanish women usually have incredibly beautiful nails. This may well be a reflection of the rich olive oil that is a mainstay of their diet. It might also date back to the fact that at one time Spanish women led such cloistered lives that they turned their attention to themselves and developed the habit of so closely grooming their nails that this preoccupation has almost become a national pastime.

As soon as our ancestors ceased using fingernails as a weapon or a tool for survival, women probably became conscious of them as another part of the body to preen and beautify. When Queen Hetepheres' tomb was opened, exquisitely wrought copper and gold manicure tools were found among the beauty implements buried with her. One of these had a sharp end for cleaning the fingernails; its opposite end was rounded for pressing back the cuticle, much like our own orange stick.

In another period, Egyptian women stained their nails with the bruised leaves of the henna plant, considering the red color an enhancement. Actually, nail polish is merely a continuation of this practice. But nowhere has the cultivation of fingernails been more impressive or carried to such lengths as by the ruling classes of China, even until fairly recent times. Four-inch fingernails were a must for the aristocracy, and a sign of rank and privilege. However, they paid for their vanity and excessive self-admiration. Imagine the grief over a broken fingernail in those days! There could be no effective patch job for a four-inch talon.

Today women find sometimes a bit of Scotch tape and a coat of polish will carry them through until their broken nail grows back to its regular length. But in the day of the privileged mandarin, a broken fingernail must have meant a lengthy period of sitting on the hand to hide the shorn member. To avoid broken nails, special sheaths were tapered to fit each nail. The coverings were formed from silver and bamboo and were themselves highly ornamental. One wonders how the Chinese were able to coax the hybrid nails into such extreme growth. It is difficult today to grow nails beyond the pad of the finger without having them peel, crack, ridge, break, or tear off.

The nutritionally rich diet of the Chinese must have held the answers. The privileged class would have had the finest and freshest fish, unrefined grains, and foods which came straight from the fields without adulteration. With this maximum nourishment, nails, of course, would grow more quickly and repair themselves more swiftly.

Even the peasant probably could have grown such nails on his own more limited, but organically pure, diet of fish, rice, and vegetables. But all that scrabbling around to earn a few cents probably wore his nails to a nubbin.

Nail growth is a condensation of keratin, an insoluble albuminous compound forming the essential ingredient of horny tissue. Within this composition is the mineral sulfur which, when broken down, yields tyrosine and leucine. These amino acids have their source in protein, taken into the body as nutrition. Going through the digestive process in the body, the protein is separated into constituent amino acids which, in turn, become the building blocks of the body.

Realizing the importance of protein if you have difficulty growing or maintaining fingernails, you might be wise to check your protein intake. Where such a shortage exists, nails can show brittleness, softness, splitting, or other evidence of nutritional shortage.

Lack of iron in the body is another cause for poor nail growth and brittleness. But this doesn't mean you should immediately start taking iron supplements. Rather, check your diet and attempt to enrich the hemoglobin with servings of liver, wheat germ, brewer's yeast, and blackstrap molasses. These easily assimilable forms of iron are preferable to inorganic iron.

Brewer's yeast is an outstanding source of iron, and as such should be included in the diet daily. An easy and palatable way of taking this rather strong-tasting powder is to dissolve it in tomato juice or other liquid. You might begin by taking a teaspoon of brewer's yeast three times a day. For the best results, slowly work up to three tablespoons a day. Your nails should reflect this increased nutrition within a short time.

Unflavored gelatin can be helpful in encouraging nail growth, too. Since it is an incomplete amino acid, it should never be taken with water alone. Rather, combine it with milk or meat broth or bouillon. Since these foods are complete proteins containing all the essential amino acids, the gelatin will then be acceptable and easily used by the body. This has to be taken daily, one tablespoon in liquid a day, to be effective.

Diet alone is not the cause of all nail problems, however. Brittle fingernails can stem from immersion in household detergents as easily as from an iron or protein deficiency. So check your household habits. When your hands come into contact with harsh detergents and other abrasive and irritating cleansers, the results can also be softened fingernails which split across the width. So damaging are some of these detergents that complete loss of the nail can sometimes occur.

Flaking of the nails also can result from bleaches and cleansers.

The wisest preventive action would be never to put your hands into either dishwater or any other solution containing a detergent action cleanser without wearing rubber gloves. This one act can assure you of strong, sturdy nails if cleansers have been the culprit.

Caution should also be used in regard to various nail hardeners on the market. There are allergenic agents in many of these products and they can create an adverse effect on a person sensitive to them. Some of the major components of nail hardeners are resin, solvent foundation, dye, and plasticizer. When used over a period of time, the nails can become brittle, with loss of tone. Covering the nails with any lacquer, whether polish or hardener, is unwise on a regular basis.

An occasional "airing" of the fingernail is advisable. During that time, perhaps every other manicure, you could remove your customary lacquer and cleanse the nails well, being sure to wash away the residue of polish remover, too. Then revitalize your nails by giving them special and needed attention in the form of a food paste instead of covering them up again with lacquer.

In this manner, the fingernail becomes a natural window for the rose-hued flesh beneath it. And if your nail care has been adequate, there is no prettier presentation of them. No lacquer can equal the loveliness of natural fingernails, reflecting and intensifying the delicate shell-pink color beneath the nail.

Time-tested suggestions advise women to apply lard or face cream beneath the nails before gardening or doing other work where deposits of grime or soil could become embedded under them. Afterward, it is easy enough to remove the fat; in this way, you avoid discoloration from mineral deposits in the soil or other accumulations. Scrub with a brush and rinse in vinegar and water or lemon juice and water to remove any final discoloration.

Buffing of the unlacquered nails has become a neglected practice for the most part. Remember the long, oval-shaped ebony or ivory buffers that used to grace every dressing table? Who uses them now? Lacquers and polishes have done away with them. And yet there is no prettier nail than the one buffed to a luster and left naturally glowing.

Cleopatra had her fingernails buffed until they shone like pearls, but you may think you haven't time for this luxury. However, as you read, watch television, or simply rest during the day, surely a few minutes could be spared for this pleasant task. If you cannot locate a buffer, use a bit of soft chamois cloth for the job. That was the material on the original buffers, anyway.

A final touch of beauty for fingernails is glossy paste. This mixture is applied directly to unlacquered nails. The alkanet root provides a subtle tinge of color. Afterward, work into a sheen by buffing the nails, which increases their luster and health. Stimulation of the subsurface will show in the quality and smoothness of the nails.

Rose Food for Fingernails

1½ ounces spermaceti
¼ ounce white wax
12 ounces sweet almond oil

2 ounces alkanet root (available from Indiana Botanic Gardens, Hammond, Ind.)
½ teaspoon rose oil

Melt the spermaceti and wax in a glass container over hot water. Beat in the sweet almond oil and alkanet root until thoroughly blended. Add the rose oil last, as the mixture begins to cool. Pour into wide-necked glass containers for easy use. Rub into clean, unpolished, dry fingernails and buff them to a high gloss.

SALT BATHS

During summer, when days are soft and warm and the body is less cluttered with clothing, the pores should be able to breathe more freely. To ensure this, the pores should be unclogged and open, and there is an excellent salt rub bath which can free the skin of flaky dead skin even as it stimulates the circulation and brings a glow of color to the body.

A sea salt rub should be performed with some vigor, but at the same time without harshness. For the grains of salt will, when wet, be softer against the skin than when dry. And the friction of grains against dead tissue will slide the stifIng scarf skin right off the body and present you with a tingling, new-as-life skin.

There are two ways to take a salt rub bath. One method is to stand in the tub with a bowl of salt to which water has been added in order to create a mushy consistency. Take a handful of the moistened salt and carefully rub all areas of the body, beginning with the neck and working downward, not missing any areas. The derrière will especially benefit from this, for any roughness will be removed. Afterward a thorough rinse under the shower will wash away the salt and dead top layer of skin.

The second method is probably the best. Stand under the shower just long enough to wet the body. Move away from the water and dip into a bowl of salt that has not been moistened. Taking up a handful, rub the body methodically from the feet up to the face.

Dip into the bowl as you require more salt. Afterward, return to the shower and rinse off. A sturdy rubbing with a towel can remove any remaining scarf skin that is ready to go.

This invigorating salt rub is a marvelous way to give your body a light peeling and allow the newer underskin to breathe. Taken once weekly, the salt rub bath can assure you of a smooth body devoid of scaliness that results from a debris-covered skin.

HAIR CONDITIONER

By now, unless you've rigged yourself out in a head covering while you gardened, swam, played, or walked in the sun, your hair may be showing the effects of too much exposure to the rays. It is during August that tragedies having to do with dull, lifeless hair usually strike. And since this has been going on since the beginning of vanity, countless means have been devised to overcome it.

First, avoid detergent shampoos. Though in the summertime you may feel that your hair seems oilier and requires more frequent shampoos, the harsh action of a detergent shampoo does more harm than good. Stick to herbal, castile, or egg shampoos for better conditioning of the hair.

In the Carribbean Islands, women use nut oils to avoid sun damage. Or they wear straw hats for protection. You might like to try a mini-tropic hair conditioner with a modern addition of liquid protein which should restore luster to dulled sun-and-water-dried hair and give it an additional bounce.

Beat 1 teaspoon of apple cider vinegar into 2 teaspoons of sesame seed oil (or any other vegetable or nut oil) and blend thoroughly. Beat in 2 tablespoons of liquid protein, which you can get from your health food store or hairdresser.

Carefully massage this solution into your dry hair and cover every area of the scalp and all the hair strands. Now comb through the hair to ensure complete coverage. Tie a plastic bag around the head and leave on for 30 minutes.

Use with an herb shampoo and rinse with 1 tablespoon of apple cider vinegar mixed into the final rinse for brunettes or the juice of half a lemon for blondes.

BREAKFAST FACIAL

A few minutes taken in the morning to apply a quickie skin feast can set the tone of your skin for several hours. It is true that external applications of nutritional ingredients alone will not perform the great benefits that a good diet will provide, but you will notice new life in your complexion if you pat on some fresh food every day.

The simpler the food chosen for a quickie morning facial, the better. In fact, it is as simple as dipping into the honey jar and patting this power-packed liquid food onto a slightly moistened face. By the time you have completed breakfast, your skin will have absorbed its quota for the moment, and you will be ready to rinse away the facial and apply your makeup.

For removing small face lines and softening and lessening deeper ones, try mixing 1 teaspoon of honey with a few drops of lemon juice. Pat onto the face and allow to remain at least 15 minutes.

SKIN STIMULANT

This is the month to fight the discomfort of too-warm days, limp hair strands, garden-damaged fingernails, and flabby skin if you haven't been exercising enough and paying close attention.

A contracting and stimulating body lotion in favor in many parts of the world uses benzoin, a resinous fluid from the trees of Sumatra and Java, and the still-vigorous crop of cucumbers which, in combination, can do much toward toning slackened skin tissues.

Use gentle, always upward circular movements when applying this or any cosmetic application to any part of the body, for you do not want to stretch the skin and further damage it. A circular movement of the fingertips combined with the astringent liquid should do much toward bringing a fresh blood supply to the area.

Grind half a cucumber and mash the pulp through gauze to extract 3 tablespoons of fresh juice. Add ¼ cup of elderflower water and 2 teaspoons of tincture of benzoin, drop by drop, shaking all the while in a capped bottle or jar.

Apply twice a day to those areas of the body which need toning.

AUGUST FOOT CARE

Continuing the plan for good foot care during the warm months, you must take note of the increasing heat and subsequent perspiration problems of the body. Perspiration in itself is nature's incredibly effective way of cooling the body surfaces. These droplets of moisture can be cleansing and refreshing to the skin. But because of bacteria on the skin and decomposition of fatty acids excreted in perspiration, unpleasant odors can result. Care, then, is required to eliminate them and regain cool comfort and scentless feet.

Changing shoes at least every day in the summer gives them a chance to dry and avoids the growth of bacteria within the shoes themselves. Open, well-fitted sandals can be another good aid for foot care. In addition, a cleansing and germicidal salt bath for the feet can do wonders in eliminating unpleasant foot odors.

For steamy, tender feet, mix a hearty handful of sea salt or iodized table salt into a basin of hot water. Dissolve the salt with the feet by moving them in a circular motion. Then relax and keep the feet immersed for 15 minutes. Dry the feet well, rubbing between the toes for extra measure. The next day, dust the feet with an unscented talcum and shake some into your shoes before putting them on.

RAW CORN MILK SKIN CLEANSER

A thirsty dry skin will drink in vitamin E when it is applied and left on overnight. The next morning, the skin feels moist, soft, and velvety in texture. By stimulating a fresh oxygen supply to the tissues, vitamin E helps the skin take on a more youthful and refreshed appearance.

Vitamin E, required by each and every cell in the body, will halt the aging process by preventing the destruction in the body of unsaturated fatty acids. A main source of this youth-preserving vitamin is unrefined vegetable oils. Corn oil would be one of these. Raw corn milk is a delicious and practical way to take this beauty vitamin fresh from its source. And August is the month to use the golden grain in every form possible.

You really get mileage from this beauty food when you drink it and use the corn milk at the same time as a complexion cleanser, without rinsing it off—really a two-in-one value. Raw corn milk is an excellent makeup remover and leaves the skin with its acid mantle intact.

Corn Milk Cocktail and Cleanser

With a sharp knife, cut the kernels off one ear of fresh corn. After the kernels are removed, run the back edge of the knife slowly up and down the ear and press out every bit of milk.

Pour this mixture into the blender and liquefy at a moderate speed. Pour into a strainer and mash through, disposing of the hulls. Two tablespoons of the raw corn milk should be enough to cleanse the face. Add a pinch of sea salt or herbal seasoning and drink the remainder.

HAIR SET FOR HUMID DAYS

Humidity runs high in August, and a coiffure which was crisp in the morning can become limp and straggly within a short time during this month. What to do to ensure curl, and/or body, during these high-humidity days?

Try an old formula dating at least from the days of the crimping iron. It is simple to prepare and requires only quince seeds and water. Simmer 1 teaspoon of quince seeds in 1 cup of water for 5 minutes; cool and strain. If this proves too thick for the hair, thin with additional water. Apply to dry hair and set as usual.

Rosemary also comes to your aid for a good hairsetting lotion which will really keep the wave in, and give body to hair even on the dampest day. Just drop a handful of rosemary leaves into a cup of water and simmer for 5 minutes; cool and strain. Use to set the hair by wetting the strands with a cotton pad dipped into the solution.

Or use skim milk as a good hair set for humid days. Instead of water, moisten the hair with the milk and proceed to set it. Do not use whole milk or you will smell like a rancid nursing baby.

To hold the hair in place once it is combed out the way you want it, pat on lemon juice, or place lemon juice and water in a 3 to 1 combination (3 teaspoons of lemon juice, 1 of water) in a squeeze spray can and spray onto the hair. This acts as a fixing agent. But don't use it too often, because of its strength, unless you dilute it with water.

RAISIN HAND CREAM
FOR ROUGHENED HANDS

No matter how thoroughly you cleanse and oil the skin, there is one trouble area which will, after the age of forty or even before, prove to need every bit of extra attention you can give it.

Hands sometimes seem to defy the best creams and lotions. When super-extra nutrition and protective applications are required, a quaint but effective cooked mixture which sounds almost good enough to eat might be the answer. Though on application it will make your hands smart, this cream is supposed to heal quickly the worst cases of chafed skin.

Mix equal quantities of lanolin, sweet butter, beeswax, and seeded chopped raisins. Simmer over a low heat until the raisins are dry but not burned. Strain into molds and cool. Rub into the hands several times a day when they are chafed and irritated. This is especially beneficial before going outdoors.

Raisins were frequently used in earlier days as a binder for other cosmetic ingredients and as a softener for the skin. Probably their rich mineral content (iron and phosphorus) created the value here.

MINT JULEP SHAMPOO

Hair showing signs of summer fatigue? Give it a quick pickup and instant nutrition with an egg mint julep shampoo. The rich sulfur content of the egg will quickly bring a gloss to dulled hair strands which are low in this mineral vital to good hair health.

Add an egg a day to your diet, and shampoo for a month on a weekly basis, or as required, with the egg mint julep shampoo. The combined external-internal approach should help restore the most lifeless hair and dispose of that end-of-the-summer appearance. The mint brings its own stimulating and refreshing qualities to add a cleansing touch to this shampoo.

To prepare the shampoo, chop a handful of fresh mint leaves and pour 1 cup of boiling water over them. Steep for 10 minutes and strain the cooled mint water. Beat 2 egg yolks to a creamy consistency and mix in the mint water. Carefully rub into scalp and every hair strand. Massage for 5 minutes, and rinse thoroughly with warm water until the water runs clear, without a trace of bubbles or foam.

ANDALUSIAN CREAM FOR OILY SKIN

The glorious sun and long summer days are here again. You garden, relax on the beach (protected from an overabundance of the powerful and destructive rays, we trust), play tennis, or just find a place to lie down and commune with nature. All that vitamin D is really marvelous for the body, and it will correct some skin problems.

Psoriasis and acne improve in the summer, and this is probably because of the vitamin D gained from exposure to the sun, though in the case of acne, the synergistic action of vitamins is thought to be responsible for this. Vitamin D improves the body's ability to assimilate calcium, and a calcium deficiency seems associated with this skin affliction.

Sometimes oily skin will worsen during the summer months, and no matter how frequently you scrub your face or sponge it with warm water, the oily patches will not go away. Attack the problem from within and without. Cut back on animal fats and switch over to lighter foods, including fresh fruits and vegetables. And try a wonderful Andalusian recipe for producing a velvety skin.

Peel an orange and a cucumber and cut 5 slices each. Force through a strainer and beat the two liquids together. Soak cotton balls in a little skim milk and apply this to a freshly washed and rinsed skin. Allow the liquid to dry. Then with a fresh cotton ball gently pat in the cucumber and orange mixture and allow it to dry on the skin also, for 20 minutes.

To rinse away, squeeze half of a fresh lemon in 2 cups of water and sponge the face thoroughly. Rinse in cold water and blot dry. Use once or twice a day, but no oftener.

SUMMER SAVORY APHRODISIAC FOR AUGUST

What hasn't been tried in the name of love to stimulate the indifferent man? Spices, fruits, herbs, and sauces of all sorts have had their advocates. One person's spice isn't necessarily another's, of course, but some of the suggestions for instant arousal that have come down to us are interesting, many times delicious, and even, on occasion, seem effective.

Summer savory, a delicately scented plant, is considered one of the finest stimulants for those short on virility or interest. So if you're uncertain of an evening, add an extra dollop of this aromatic herb to a bland salad.

For the salad itself, you might try a combination of watercress, with its calcium, phosphorus, and iron; apple, with its sulfur and magnesium; and summer savory with its own mystique of volatile oil which acts as a tonic. If you feel really reckless, you might want to take a bath with a splash of the oil in your tub, for additional insurance. According to herbalists, summer savory strengthens body tissues, so it could rightly be considered a double agent, acting both from within and without.

Add the salad to an energy-boosting meal and determine whether the herbalists are right in their prescription for a savory evening.

EXERCISES FOR THE SHOULDERS

The prettiest figure can be spoiled by a rounded mound of flesh rising between the shoulder blades. In fact, even this one disfigurement can destroy the image of a beautiful person. First impressions are, without your actually being aware of it, based on body framework. If you don't have good straight posture, all your other attributes diminish accordingly.

Drooping shoulders suggest a weariness and age which may have nothing to do with years. In time, the casual carriage of youth, if not corrected, turns into a middle-aged slump which can give a tired appearance to a twenty-year-old.

The following exercises for trimming away excess fat which develops in untoned shoulder areas are always successful if practiced daily. In addition to restoring good body lines, the movements are invigorating and restorative. Relieved of their heavy burden of unneeded and dangerous fat, the shoulders will lift up to a straighter position.

Kneel on the floor with the elbows placed directly in front of the bent knees, the forepart of the arm and the palms flat before you. Move the knees backward about one foot. Take a deep breath and rise upward with your feet held flat on the floor, the knees assuming a straight position. Hold the elbows on the floor, with the body weight on the arms and toes. Slowly raise the head as high as possible. Exhale and return the knees to the floor.

It is lifting up your head while the body is in its jackknifed position that actually benefits the shoulder area, by strengthening and toning it. The complete pull on the upper center back area works at excess flesh and flabby muscles. The upward movement of the head while the arms and legs support the body also brings a fresh blood supply to the face, stimulating it for a beauty flush. The chest area is stretched in this slanted position and a more normal breathing pattern is created. Altogether, this is a multi-purpose exercise, benefiting, as it does, so many parts of the body.

BREAKFASTS FOR AUGUST

❧⊰⊱❧

Fresh plums
Wheat germ, soya grains, and raisins
Herbal tea

Cantaloupe
Omelet with chives and parsley
Whole grain bread
Herbal tea

Bananas in milk
Rice flour pancakes (recipe on p. 21) with plum sauce
Herbal tea

Honeydew melon
Potato pancakes (recipe on p. 238)
Herbal tea

Bowl of grapes
Poached eggs on corn cakes (recipe on p. 213)
Herbal tea

Pears stewed with honey
Granola (recipe on p. 21)
Herbal tea

Grape juice
Oatmeal and currants
Herbal tea

LUNCHES FOR AUGUST

Cold beet borscht (recipe on p. 93)
Garbanzo salad (recipe on p. 46)
Yogurt

Chilled fruit soup*
Tuna salad
Yogurt

Raw salad bowl
Peanut butter and sesame seed sandwiches with apple slices
Yogurt

Spinach, lettuce, and cabbage salad
Squash griddle cakes (recipe on p. 70)
Yogurt

Cream of broccoli soup with nasturtium buds (recipe on p. 165)
Nut butter sandwiches (recipe on p. 43)
Yogurt

Corn soup (recipe on p. 166)
Raw shoestring salad with beets, peppers, and carrots
Yogurt

Fresh tomato soup*
Rolled oatcakes (recipe on p. 69) with mung sprouts
Yogurt

DINNERS FOR AUGUST

Cashew and vegetable dinner*
Brown rice
Beets in lemon butter

Sardines and parsleyed potatoes
Pimento coleslaw
String beans

Giblets and brown rice with chrysanthemum petals
Beets
Shredded and steamed cabbage

Sautéed brains with tomato sauce
Potatoes in jacket
Chard

Baked cheese omelet with marigold petals*
Parsley minted potatoes
String beans

Lentil loaf (recipe on p. 22) or soy rice
Parsnips
Turnip, mustard, or collard greens

Tomatoes stuffed with soya beans
Corn
Kohlrabi

RECIPES FOR AUGUST

Chilled Fruit Soup

2 tablespoons arrowroot	1 apple, chopped
2 cups water	1 cup cherries
1 cup fresh orange juice	2 tablespoons lemon juice
1 cup strawberries	honey to taste

Mix the arrowroot in enough water to make a thin paste. Put remaining water and orange juice in a saucepan and heat. Stir in the arrowroot and cook until thickened. Add other ingredients and simmer 5 minutes. Dilute with additional fruit juice according to consistency desired. May be served hot or cold.

Fresh Tomato Soup

2 cups chopped, peeled tomatoes	2 teaspoons olive oil
	1 teaspoon minced onion
2 leaves minced sweet basil	sea salt to season

Place all ingredients into blender and blend well. Serve cold.

Cashew and Vegetable Dinner

raw cashew nuts

vegetable oil

curry powder

1 clove finely chopped garlic

salt

½ lb. fresh string beans

enough milk to moisten

Over low flame, cover bottom of an iron pan with a single layer of raw cashew nuts. Dry roast them and stir to keep them from being scorched. When they are roasted, pour them out into a bowl. Pour enough oil to cover the bottom of the iron pan up to ⅛ of an inch. Maintain a low flame. Brown a clove of finely chopped garlic, then stir in 1 tablespoon of curry powder. Pour the nuts back into the pan and stir. Cook for 2 or 3 minutes and add ½ pound of fresh string beans. Stir nuts, beans, etc., until coated. Pour milk over the entire mixture, add salt, and simmer for 20 to 30 minutes.

(Cabbage, broccoli, or other suitable green vegetable can be substituted for the string beans.)

Baked Cheese Omelet with Marigold Petals

1½ cups milk

3 tablespoons cornmeal

sea salt

2 cups grated Swiss cheese

3 eggs, beaten separately

¼ cup marigold petals

Scald milk in top of double boiler. Slowly beat in cornmeal mixed with salt and stir until the mixture thickens. Remove from heat and blend in cheese. Allow to cool a bit and beat very slowly into the egg yolks. Fold in the stiffly beaten whites and marigold petals and pour into an oiled casserole. Bake at 425 degrees until golden brown, around 25 minutes.

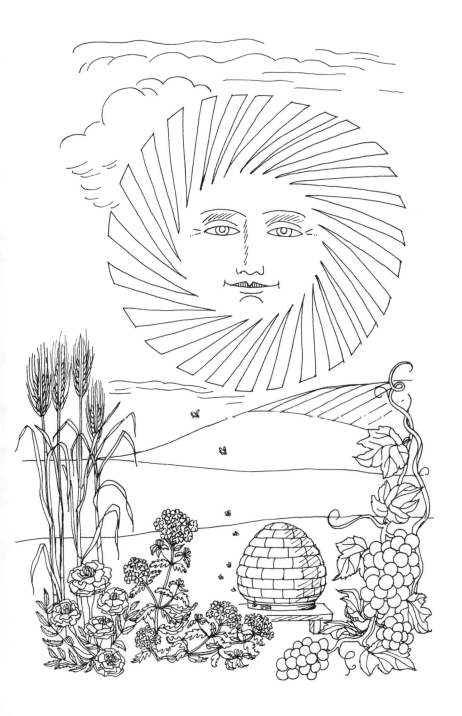

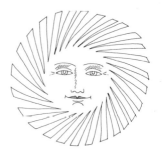

September

Earth is all in splendor drest;
Queenly fair, she sits at rest,
While in the deep, delicious day
Dreams its happy life away.

   Margaret Sangster: "An Autumn Day"

Called variously Autumn Month, Barley Month, and Holy Month, the French calendar prefers Fruit Month. And the French were probably thinking of the delicious Anjou pears that turn golden on the branches before they are picked and brought to market. Barley can be used in soups and as a facial wash, and since this is its month according to early harvest calendars, plan to add its soothing alkaline properties to your diet and beauty care.

Add also the various nuts that come upon the market this month. But at the same time, don't neglect the last of the flowers. Wear them in your hair, put them on your salads, and brew them into softening potions for your complexion, strengthening it for the months of cold weather to come. To be thorough, reach backward for summer's last wealth even as you lean forward toward the harvests of fall.

CLEANSING OF THE FALL SKIN

September brings with it a desire to correct the indulgences of summer—of time in the sun which seemed to call for frequent showers taken more for refreshment than for body scouring. And how delightful it was to splash water across the face and feel the freshness. But now you look more intently in the mirror, and perhaps see pores which need cleansing because of the easy summer care program.

To use soap or not to use soap as a facial cleaner remains a controversial issue among many women. There are those who speak of a favorite soap they have used for years, and whose skin remains firm, clear, and unclogged. Others will disagree and show faces just as clear with skin as delicate and finely textured as the soap users.

There are dangers to washing with soap, and avoiding its use at least on the face and neck areas seems indicated in certain instances. First, if your soap doesn't have a pH acid factor, then you are using an alkaline type cleanser which robs your skin of its protective acid mantle and leaves it exposed to bacterial invasion.

For safety's sake, purchase Squibb's Nitrazine paper in a pharmacy and keep it on hand to test any new soap or cosmetic you use. Most soaps test alkaline, a deep purple on nitrazine paper, and are thus possibly harmful to the skin and certainly not protective of it.

In contrast, dip a small strip of the nitrazine paper into a solution of rosemary infusion. The paper remains a bright yellow, indicating an excellent cleanser for the skin, though better for oily and normal skins than for dry. Rinse the skin afterward, to avoid staining.

To avoid the possible dangers of a too-alkaline soap, there are several possibilities in addition to searching out the acid-based soaps.

If you insist on using the usual market type soap, you can add a teaspoon or so of apple cider vinegar to a pint of water and keep it for a final rinse, blotting the face dry afterward. This will help restore the acid mantle native to the skin.

To avoid the use of soaps altogether for deep facial skin cleansing, you can use fresh milk as an entirely satisfactory means. Dip small cotton pads into the milk and gently rub in rotating movements, always upward, over the face and neck area. For the best results, warm the milk slightly. If your skin is dry, beat in a few drops of vegetable oil. Discard the cotton pads frequently, and use fresh ones as needed.

RUM SHAMPOO FOR NORMAL HAIR

The French are very knowledgeable about caring for their hair. Seldom if ever do you see a Frenchwoman with flyaway, tangled, or limp strands. The average Frenchwoman cherishes her hair, guards it, and lavishes her closest attention on its care.

A favorite shampoo, of even hairdressers themselves in Paris, is the rum and egg combination. Avoiding soaps, the Frenchwoman with limp locks can coax the finest performance from dull hair with the rum and egg mixture.

Rum Toddy Shampoo

¼ cup rum   1 egg yolk

Beat together thoroughly for several minutes. Apply to dry hair that has first been well brushed to rid it of dust and loose dandruff. Massage into the hair for 5 minutes, gently stimulating the scalp with the fingertips. Cover all areas, then rinse under warm water for several minutes until the water runs clear and unclouded. Towel dry or to the degree of dampness you need to set your hair.

BAGHDAD HAND PASTE

Swimming in chlorinated water, sun exposure, and gardening, all cherished preoccupations of summer, have by now left their marks on your hands. Time to put away the summer's pleasures and pastimes, get the body winter-worthy, and concentrate on corrective measures.

Rough-textured hands respond dramatically to a paste of honey and almonds. The recipe comes from Baghdad, by way of one of Billy Rose's fabulous Diamond Horseshoe girls. Dolly married a handsome Baghdadi and went to live in his palace. This showgirl was a Texas beauty with no problems except dry hands, which had kept her constantly scouting for better hand creams and more effective lotions.

Her problems ended in Baghdad. Her mother-in-law also was captivated by this spirited girl, even though Dolly refused to accept the traditional veil worn by wives in that part of the world. (Instead, she took the long, golden chain that held the veiled headdress in place and wore it as a necklace which clicked briskly as she waltzed around the castle.) To signal her acceptance, her mother-in-law prepared a mixture for her, and this flamboyant rebel finally had her hands made beautiful.

Baghdad Hand Paste

8 ounces honey
4 ounces almond meal

1 tablespoon egg yolk
8 ounces sweet almond oil

Heat the honey slightly and beat into the almond meal. Add the egg yolk and knead together. Slowly add the almond oil, a few drops at a time, and continue kneading until a paste has formed. Dolly added a sprinkle of rose oil to the paste, as the oil is easily obtained in Baghdad. You may add perfume or not. Use daily.

THE DRY BATH

Wouldn't it be nice to have a body as sleek and polished as the smoothest marble? To be able to run your hands down the surface of your skin and feel no bumps, calloused protuberances, or roughened areas?

One splendid way to remove superficial roughness and dispose of dead and clogging cellular waste is with a luffa mitt. Long used in Europe and the Orient as a necessary part of external body upkeep, this naturally grown fiber has the ability to hone the skin to a sleekness which cannot be achieved with the usual washcloth.

Incredibly rough in texture, the luffa is actually not as harsh in use as it appears to be. Running it lightly across the body surfaces, it loosens and flakes off that tissue that no longer has life, and if left, only clogs the skin and gives it a coarse texture and appearance. Do not use force or great effort with the luffa. Its spidery-webbed texture makes that unnecessary.

Though there are a variety of friction mitts on the market, including plastic ones, buy only the natural vegetable luffa, coming from the gourd family. In fact, if you plant the right gourd seed, you can grow your own luffa mitt. Another good method of dry bathing is with a natural bristle brush, which will serve the same purpose as the luffa. But it must be a natural bristle instead of nylon, as nylon does not have the resiliency of the bristle.

Start with your feet and, using circular movements, gradually work upward on the body, avoiding only the face and breast area. Work gently in spiraling movements until you have ended the dry friction bath with a gentle rubbing of the neck areas.

If you would like to lessen the friction of the dry glove, try sprinkling a solution made from 2 tablespoons of rosemary leaves steeped in 1 cup of hot water, then strained. This softens the contact of the luffa and at the same time acts as a disinfectant and antiseptic.

The luffa is sold in European shops as an aid in breaking down and redistributing fat deposits on the hips and other parts of the body. It will certainly help bring about better muscle tone in the body and a greater elasticity to the skin.

After a body brushing lasting at least 5 minutes, it is a good idea to take a shower to wash away the flaked and dead skin loosened on the body surfaces by the dry scrubbing. Towel dry and, if you would like the luxury, apply an almond milk body lotion (see recipe in December).

VERBENA WASH FOR THE SKIN

One of the last flowers to go and one that is still blooming in shades of purple and pink this month is the verbena. When brewed into a facial tea, it acts as a stimulant for the skin. Lemony in scent, the verbena used daily as a last splash on the face instead of plain water adds its own toning and fragrant qualities to a leftover summer complexion.

Verbena Wash

Place a tablespoon of flower heads and leaves, rinsed in cool water, in a cup. Pour boiling water over them, cover, and steep for 10 minutes. Use when completely cool, and blot the face dry. Do not rinse off.

At the same time you use the verbena face wash, incorporate the sedative effects of the dried flower petals in a tea sweetened with honey to offset its slightly bitter tang. Be at peace with a calming tisane, or cup of the brew, as you derive benefits from the soothing lotion and realize you are profiting from the flower in more ways than one.

Collect and dry as many of these fragrant blossoms as you can for use later in the year, when a flower wash and soothing cup of tea can cheer a long fall day.

BARLEY BEAUTY

Since September is barley month, eat the pearly grain in soups and pat it onto the face and neck for good skin toning. Internally, this old-fashioned and highly nutritious food contributes to good blood circulation and soothes the agitated mind that is restless and wandering. Rich in niacin, one of the B vitamins, barley's frequent inclusion in the diet can help prevent skin outbreaks and contribute to overall health. The following drink is a beverage used by the Queen of England, and her exquisite complexion certainly says much for its use.

Barley Water

2½ quarts boiling water   honey to taste
½ cup barley   rinds from 2 lemons
6 oranges (free of spray or
artificial coloring)

Pour boiling water over the barley and simmer over low heat for
1 hour. Squeeze the oranges, set juice aside, and reserve rinds.
Strain the water from the cooked barley into a bowl and add the
honey and rinds from the oranges and lemons. Allow to stand
until cold. Remove the rinds and add the fruit juice. Refrigerate
and drink as desired.

SKIN BLEACHING

Though warm days may linger on in Indian summer style, fall
greets us with the coming of September. In the South, the whistle
of the cotton gin summoning the wagon-high loads of fluffy cotton
bolls toward their processing operation into bales begins. West-
ward, the cactus thrusts forth rampant coloring of delicate red
and yellow blossoms over their spiky plants. To the east and north,
the birds fly south toward palmettos and moss, and women turn
ritually toward darker colors, as though satiated with the pastel
coloring of an abundant summer.

Darkened skin tones, however, do not go as well with the more
somber clothing preferred in some areas of the country. In addition, tans are fading, leaving sallow skin tones behind. Without the
spark of color in your cheeks, fall's deeper tones do nothing for
your appearance. Thus, it is time to make ready for this season,

to clear away mixed skin coloring, to clean hardened elbows, and to restore your own basic skin tones.

Mix the juice of ½ fresh lemon with an equal amount of sweet almond oil. Massage into the face, neck, elbows, and knees. Allow the covering to remain for 15 minutes. Remove by gently scrubbing with a textured washcloth. Rinse in warm, then cool, water and blot dry. Repeat as needed. One treatment is seldom sufficient. But this month and the next should see an end to leftover sallowness if you start now to treat these uneven skin tones.

SPANISH WHEAT PASTE
FOR IRRITATED SKIN

In Spain, they toss the wheat high into the sky, and as it drops earthward, the chaff is caught by the wind and spun away across the newly mown fields. The wheat grain piles up as the ancient winnowing process is repeated, and mounds of the golden grain glow in the brilliant plains sunlight.

From this wheat comes the food for the year and a valued cosmetic item. The fact that it never rains on the plains in Spain emphasizes the harshness of the Avila region, where grain is used in a valued beauty preparation.

A favorite method for soothing irritated cheeks, whether from an allergic reaction or an overdose of wind or sun, is a paste made from plains wheat which nourishes and heals at the same time.

Soak 2 tablespoons of whole wheat flour in enough warm milk to make a loose paste. Beat the mixture smooth and allow it to soften for 10 minutes before spreading it over the irritated area. After it dries, rinse away in warm, then cool, water. Gently rub in a thin film of oil and blot away the excess. Apply the paste daily until the area is without blemish.

MARIGOLD SKIN SOOTHER
AND CLEANSER

A delicious and delightful cosmetic food, marigold, the flower of the sun, provides advantages as a food and when used externally. Legend says the sun's power is caught in the golden-petaled blossoms and its strength is released in complexion creams and washes for the hair. Soothing to burning feet, marigold cream is equally helpful as a skin cleanser. *Calendula officinalis* is the older variety of marigold that is recommended for these recipes rather than the recently developed hybrids and strains.

When made into an infusion or tea, marigold used as a lotion is an excellent wash for excessively oily skins and blotched complexions.

Marigold Lotion for Oily Skin

Pull the petals from a handful of marigold heads. Drop them into a cup of warm milk. Simmer for 5 minutes, strain, and cool before using. This lotion does not have to be left on, but can be used as any cleansing lotion by gently rubbing away with cotton pads and then rinsing the face with warm and then cool water. Refrigerate when not in use.

Marigold Cream

Heat 2 tablespoons of almond nut butter (purchase in a health food shop or make your own). Mix in 1 tablespoon of macerated marigold petals and blend together. To use, apply the paste to a face moistened with warm water. Rub gently into the skin and allow to remain for a minimum of 30 minutes.

Almond Nut Butter

⅓ cup sweet almond oil   ½ cup almond meal
⅓ cup lemon juice

Beat the sweet almond oil and lemon juice together and blend in the almond meal. If more liquid is required to create a spreadable consistency, add a bit of rose water, elderflower water, orange flower water, or mineral water.

MARIGOLD RINSE FOR THE HAIR

The golden-headed marigold should be restored to the position it occupied during the Middle Ages. Enriching both salads and stews with its pungent, exotic scent, this flower that blossoms on into the first days of September serves equally well as a hair rinse for light hair. Marsh-gold, or marygold, as it has also been known, follows the sun as it travels across the sky and drinks in the life-giving rays all day, much as does the sunflower.

Steeped in vinegar, marigolds have been used to relieve aching gums. But medieval maidens prized it most for its yellow coloring which they used as a hair rinse for blond hair, to retain lightness or camouflage drabbing. For better coloring qualities, again use the *Calendula officinalis* or you may not get good results.

To gain greater benefits from marigolds, gather the tightly clustered heads and sprinkle the petals loosely on clean tissue paper and allow them to dry in some airy place until all the moisture disappears from the petals.

Drop ½ cup of the dried petals into 2 cups of boiling water and steep for 10 minutes. Strain and use as a final hair rinse, catching the liquid in a basin and pouring it over the hair several times. Do not rinse out, and for even greater benefits, sit in the sun to dry your hair, fluffing it out from time to time so the sun can reach every area.

OLIVE NIGHT CREAM

When you are trying through daily exercise to regain the elasticity of skin that was lost to the summer sun or to the insistent play of years, you can help to bring this about by restoring moisture and plumping the cells a bit in external applications.

Olive night cream is a satiny mixture which can bring a velvety texture and more vibrant smoothness to a lined, drying skin. Spanish and Italian women can usually be envied their smooth skin, and surely the frequent use of this rich, nourishing oil supports that skin.

Mix together 3 tablespoons of lanolin, 2 tablespoons of virgin olive oil, and 1 tablespoon of rose water, orange blossom water, or mineral water. Heat to a liquid consistency in a glass custard cup or small jar set in a pan of hot water.

Apply nightly to a freshly scrubbed face with no traces of cleansing cream. Bathe the face in the morning in warm water without soap, then splash with an herbal rinse or plain cool water. Fennel tea is a good rinse after the olive night cream.

HONEY FOR SOFTENING LINES

The skin that is soft and elastic is the skin that will wear well, conceal age to a great degree, and be delightful to make up. Leathery, dowdy skin defies attempts to conceal, and to practice successfully any makeup artistry, there has to be a basis to work on.

Honey is one of the cosmetic miracles of all time, which can help return a damaged skin surface to a fresh and finely textured complexion. Anyone with roughened, coarse-toned skin can usually feel with a touch of the fingers a difference after using honey as a softener. The time required for this transformation varies, but within a short time there should be a great improvement and an ageless rather than an aged look.

Anemic skin can also benefit from this mineral-rich food which stimulates and softens at the same time. Honey alone is a fine nourishing cream for the fatigued skin. Combined with other life-giving foods, other qualities are added, according to the ingredients used. You can have a different honey facial every day of the week and ensure a constant and wide-range skin feeding which will moisturize, soften, enliven, invigorate, and at the same time, lessen the fine line wrinkling of the face.

Honey Facial

1. Mix 1 teaspoon of dark honey with 1 teaspoon of fresh cream. (Top milk, coffee cream, or heavy whipping cream will do. Do *not* use prewhipped aerosol fluff or milk "foods.") For dry or normal skin.

2. Mix 1 teaspoon of honey, ½ teaspoon of egg yolk, and a few drops of lemon juice. For dry, flaky skin.

3. Blend together 1 teaspoon honey with 1 teaspoon unbeaten egg white. For dry or normal skin.

4. Beat 1 teaspoon of honey with ½ teaspoon of corn oil. For normal or dry skin.

5. Blend 1 teaspoon of honey with 1 teaspoon of fresh orange juice. For colorless skin.

6. Beat together 1 teaspoon honey and 1 teaspoon of mashed banana. For normal or oily skin.

7. Beat together 1 teaspoon honey and 1 teaspoon of red wine. For pale, anemic skin.

SOVEREIGNE WATER TO STAY YOUNG

The virtues of sovereign waters are formidable, according to its sixteenth-century originator. John Partridge suggested taking a gallon of good Gascoine wine and adding 1 teaspoon of the following spicy ingredients. (As for the wine, you could try a good burgundy in lieu of the Gascoine.)

ginger   cloves
cinnamon   mace
nutmeg   anise seeds
caraway seeds   fennel seeds

John's formula says, "Take sage, minte, red roses, thyme, camomile and lavender, of every one of them a handful." Beat the spices (listed above) small, he suggests. I suggest using powdered spices, or popping whole spices into an electric grinder or blender to pulverize them.

Bruise the herbs and toss with the spices into the wine and let stand for 12 hours. Stir thoroughly from time to time to mix all the powerful scents and tastes together.

Distill the liquid and, according to an abbreviated description of the original commentary, you have a spirit that preserveth one greatly. So much so that according to John Partridge, "It will preserve him in good liking and shall make one seeme young very long."

If you do not own a water still, it is easy enough to improvise one to use in this formula. Slip a rubber tube over the spout of a tea kettle containing the mixture. Place the tube in a shallow pan of ice cubes and insert the other end of the tube into a glass where the moisture will drop after the kettle has been heated enough to produce condensed steam.

GRAPE WASH

The fruits of all the land are bursting forth in one last offering. Corn is still heaped in piles at roadside stands, and the golden pear and jewel-toned grapes are offerings to make the heart sing in gratitude. No matter how automated our food industry becomes or how sterile the preparations for commercial meals, there will always be that richness of nature that makes our primitive and knowledgeable spirit respond to the harvest with gratitude.

Iron-rich purple grapes are indeed a beauty potion to offer the face. Green grapes contain less iron, but are valuable as a face wash and feast. Alkaline by nature, the grape, both green and purple, has been considered a help in some skin disorders when included in the diet often enough. So in September eat the fruit and wear it and thereby benefit with an internally cleansed and strengthened body, and new skin tone from its supplies of vitamins A, B, C, and rich mineral content of potassium, magnesium, sulfur, and phosphorus.

For a facial wash, drop a few grapes into the blender and reduce them to a pulp. Strain through gauze and dab onto the face from time to time, allowing each application to dry before patting on more liquid.

APHRODISIAC FOR SEPTEMBER

The Romans called it reinforcing sexuality, or giving a natural inclination a delightful boost. Like preparing a Wine of Love.

In France, the drink of love could be considered champagne, and after a glass or two, its effervescent bubbling does seem to quicken the interest. But overenthusiastic drinking of champagne can sometimes leave a headache, whereas the Wine of Love seems to ease you into and out of the evening with only pleasant memories. Anyway, the following is supposed to be a gentle though effective means of stimulation to the jaded or the reluctant.

Wine of Love

Combine 1 quart of sherry with 2 tablespoons of sugar, the juice of 2 oranges, plus 1 teaspoon of grated orange rind. Add to this 1 teaspoon of nutmeg and ½ teaspoon of cinnamon. Bring just to a simmer and serve warm.

WAIST EXERCISES

Summer's indulgences are behind us now, but some of the results can linger on if we dug too deeply into refreshing bowls of ice cream and tempting portions of strawberry shortcake. September is a good time to buckle down and whittle away at these extra inches so that fall clothes will fit smoothly and comfortably. You can effectively restore your figure to that exquisite trimness that allowed you to walk freely and bend and stretch with ease. There are several good exercises for narrowing the waist, reducing the flabby roll of flesh around the middle, and generally correcting the summer's excesses.

An exercise which literally grinds the extra inches away can be performed standing with the hands placed on the hips in a supportive fashion.

Stand erect with the palms on the hips. Very slowly move from right to left, completing a small circle with the upper part of your body as you sway around with your feet flat on the floor. Without stopping, continue the rolling movement, keeping the knees straight and the toes pointed slightly outward for good body balance.

As you gain physical flexibility and sureness of movement, you will find the swing of your upper torso increases, and with it smoothness of performance.

Reverse the swing from the right to the left and repeat.

Another exercise is done lying flat on your back on the floor with your arms clasped behind your head. Slowly raise your knees as close to your chest as possible. Very slowly turn your knees toward the floor to your left, while turning your head to the right. Very slowly, return to the center, knees still touching your chest, and turn toward the right, turning your head to the left. Continue this twisting movement several times, or as long as it is comfortable.

BREAKFASTS FOR SEPTEMBER

⟜⧈⟊

Date nut drink*
Whole grain toast with eggs and mushrooms
Herbal tea

Melon
Baked eggplant slices with soft-boiled egg
Herbal tea

Apple juice
Rice flour pancakes (recipe on p. 21) with grape jelly
Herbal tea

Bananas and wheat germ
Poached eggs on cornmeal chapaties (recipe on p. 23)
Herbal tea

Stewed pears
Buckwheat groats
Herbal tea

Stewed apples with barley pancakes*
Herbal tea

Fresh grape juice or bottled Concord grape juice
Brown rice and raisins
Herbal tea

LUNCHES FOR SEPTEMBER

Potato and leek soup
Salad of chard, spinach, watercress, and onion
Yogurt

Oatmeal soup*
Raw vegetable bowl
Yogurt

Corn soup (recipe on p. 166)
Salad bowl of raw turnip slices, carrots, and celery
Yogurt

Barley soup
Corn cakes with wheat germ*
Yogurt

Vegetable broth
Carrot and pineapple salad
Yogurt

Frseh tomato soup (recipe on p. 189)
Nut and fruit salad
Yogurt

Finger fruit salad with cottage cheese and yogurt dip*
Sprout bread and nut butter (recipe on p. 45)

Chef salad with cheese strips
Avocado sandwich*
Yogurt

DINNERS FOR SEPTEMBER

Egg Foo Yung*
Carrots with mint
Brown rice and minced green onions

Carrot patties*
Cheese potatoes
Cabbage salad

Chicken livers and mushrooms
Zucchini and tomato casserole

Vegetable loaf*
Mung sprouts with onions
Steamed beets with grated lemon peel and oil

Broiled fish
Beets and beet tops
Parsnips

Cottage cheese burgers*
Jerusalem artichokes
Tomatoes and green onions with lemon, oil, and parsley dressing

Kidneys en brochette
Rice
Tomato and onion salad

RECIPES FOR SEPTEMBER

Date Nut Drink

¼ cup sunflower seeds
4 dates
milk or 2 tablespoons soya milk
    powder

honey to sweeten
2 cups water

Grind seeds in blender. Add the remaining ingredients and liquefy.

Barley Pancakes

1 cup barley flour
2 teaspoons baking powder
¼ teaspoon sea salt

2 teaspoons vegetable oil
1 beaten egg
1 cup water

Beat ingredients together, adding additional water if a thinner batter is desired. Bake on hot griddle.

Oatmeal Soup

1 cup minced onion
1 cup minced celery
1 cup sliced mushrooms
1 cup steel-cut oatmeal
1 teaspoon sea salt

4 tablespoons vegetable oil
2 bay leaves
¼ cup minced parsley
1 pint water

Cook onion, celery, and mushrooms in oil until soft. Add oatmeal and brown slightly. Add remaining ingredients and simmer for 30 minutes. Remove bay leaves and serve.

Corn Cakes

1 cup corn flour	1 cup sour milk
½ cup wheat germ	½ cup sour cream
½ teaspoon baking soda	2 tablespoons salad oil
½ teaspoon baking powder	1 beaten egg
½ teaspoon sea salt	1 tablespoon honey

Combine all ingredients and bake on hot griddle.

Finger Fruit Salad

fresh pineapple cut in sticks	fresh coconut sticks
papaya strips	bananas dipped in lemon juice
peach wedges	and sliced

Pour over the fruit a dressing made of honey and lemon juice.

Avocado Sandwich

Mash 1 avocado to a fine pulp and add 2 teaspoons of lemon juice. Mix in ½ mashed garlic clove with 2 tablespoons sour cream and beat all together. Spread on whole grain bread.

Egg Foo Yung

4 beaten eggs
1 cup bean sprouts
¼ cup chopped water chestnuts

¼ cup minced green onion
1 celery stalk, minced

Mix together and allow 1 large tablespoon of the mixture for each pattie. Brown in oil in heavy skillet.

Carrot Patties

1 cup ground carrots
½ cup ground sunflower seeds
1 cup ground almonds

1 beaten egg yolk
1 teaspoon summer savory
¼ cup pecan meal

Mix first five ingredients together and flatten balls of the mixture into the ground pecan meal. Serve uncooked.

Vegetable Loaf

1 eggplant
1 minced tomato
1 minced onion
2 stalks minced celery
4 tablespoons salad oil
1 beaten egg
1 tablespoon sour cream

½ cup whole grain bread
    crumbs
2 tablespoons wheat germ
1 clove minced garlic
sea salt
2 leaves sweet basil
½ teaspoon oregano

Put peeled eggplant through the grinder and sauté with other vegetables in 4 tablespoons oil. Cool by pouring into bowl. Mix in remaining ingredients. Bake at 350 degrees for 30 minutes.

Cottage Cheese Burgers

2 cups cottage cheese
1 minced onion
½ cup wheat germ

½ cup whole wheat crumbs
1 tablespoon salad oil

Mix together and allow 1 heaping tablespoon for each burger.
Bake at 325 degrees on an oiled cookie sheet for 30 minutes.

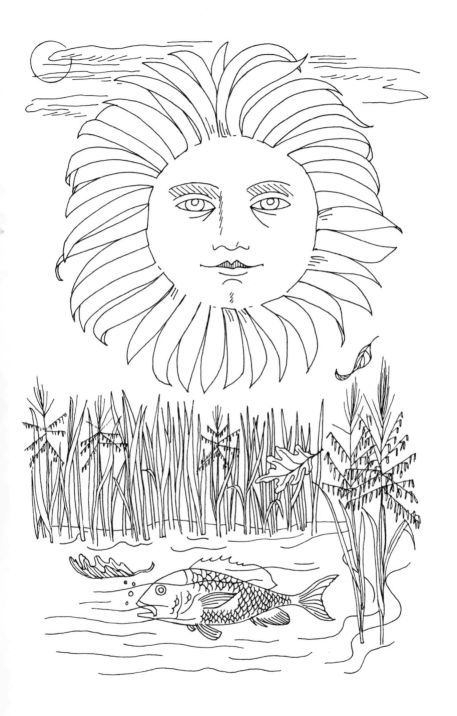

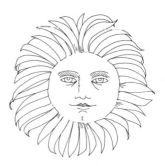

October

*The sweet calm sunshine of October,
now
Warms the low spot; upon its grassy
mould
The purple oak-leaf falls; the birchen
bough
Drops its bright spoil like arrow-heads
of gold.*

William Cullen Bryant: "October, 1866"

With the tenth month of the year, full of its gold and mellow days, comes a sense of shortening time. All that is good we have had in the past months. But still, in richness, this month offers itself as Wine Month, Winter Full Moon, and Time of Vintage. With the harvesting of the grains during this time, even the drinks took on a happy sound in A Tankard of October, which was a goodly strong brew of ale for those who had harvested well, and now could sit back and view their bounty, knowing that all would be well for the less friendly months ahead when a fulfilled nature retrenches and rests.

Stock should be taken of yourself, no less than the land. It's time to remove leftover skin discolorations which haven't yet responded fully to less sun exposure, to munch a freshly picked apple, and to lather a slice of it into your hungry skin. Time to prepare a protective paste for hands which don't take kindly to cooler days, and to take deep breaths of crisp, clear air. Beauty breathing will teach you to handle your emotions better by bringing great new supplies of oxygen to your body. At the same time, this freshening of the blood supply will cleanse the inner body and be reflected in clearer skin tones.

THIGH EXERCISES

The real leg-stretching days are over for many, with this month's return to offices and desk sitting. Full acknowledgment that fall is upon us and that October means closing the windows and sitting for long hours with only a memory of summer's outdoor pleasures can result in disastrous figure problems unless you take preventive measures.

Perhaps indoor exercise isn't as exciting as long striding walks down the curve of a beach or splendid hikes through the woods. But the need for exercise continues, the rewards are great, and you will swing into October and the months to come sleek and agile if you spare just a few minutes a day to keep intact your trim summer figure.

There is no doubt that leg complaints and problems have increased as our sedentary lifestyle has evolved. Men and women once had trim, sturdy legs which carried them gracefully through their days, but this is not always true now. Thighs bulge and, for the most part, are too heavy, in addition to being uncomfortable to live with.

Yet to these limbs we are indebted for mobility, and a chance to live free, as anyone who can move like the wind is free.

Office work or work that confines you to a chair for the greater portion of the day, is one of the main culprits in leg trouble. The very position of sitting and having the rim of the chair press into the underpart of the leg just beneath the knee joint is detrimental to good circulation.

Merely crossing the legs with the underthigh supported by the lower thigh can create undesirable effects by limiting blood circulation. You become aware of this when, after sitting in this position, you find you must switch legs back and forth as they grow increasingly fatigued.

While changing legs will help by removing the pressure on the blood vessels and thereby the constriction, it would be even better not to cross your legs at all. Instead, cross them at the ankles where the weight is less.

To combat leg stress if you must sit for long periods, try to get up and walk around as often as possible. In addition, do daily leg-stretching exercises to take care of any flab which might develop from long hours of sitting. The slantboard can perform near miracles in restoring tired legs. A fifteen-minute slantboard rest at any time of weariness probably gives better results than an hour's nap, because it exerts a counter-pull on aching legs and affords the veins in the legs a chance to rid themselves of the heavy blood flow.

If practiced daily, these exercises will restore muscle tone, strengthen the thighs, and relieve the cramping that results from poor circulation.

Wear loose clothing and no shoes. Sitting on the floor with your legs straight before you, bend the right knee and draw it toward your chest. Reach forward with both hands and grasp the foot from both sides. Very slowly straighten the knee completely and extend your leg upward on an angle from the body. Hold your back as straight as possible and avoid tumbling backward. Maintain the position as long as is comfortable, then slowly lower your leg to its original position. Repeat with the other leg.

Another exercise requires you to take a seated position on the floor with your legs stretched out before you. Keeping the knees stiff, allow your feet to make alternate paddling movements, up and down, without the heels ever leaving the floor. The toes will be reaching for the floor but, obviously, will not touch it. The pull on the calves can be felt immediately. And the toning of the legs is excellent in this movement. In fact, you will feel the pull all the way to your thighs.

SOOTHING BATHS

There's nothing nicer than a good bath for tired muscles reaccustoming themselves to the strictures of cooler weather. I often wonder, though, whether it was easier or more agreeable to take a bath in pre-plumbing days when someone else heated the water and filled the tub and all you had to do was sink into it after a busy autumn day. Somehow, baths taken then always sound so elegant and splendid. And yet, what could be a richer and more luxurious feeling than turning on the faucet to the exact temperature down to the *nth* degree in a modern tub?

The only thing I envy those earlier bathers is the incredibly low cost of some of the beauty ingredients available then. And alas, they are hardly obtainable now, unless you scout around or prepare your own. Take, for example, rose water, which could be bought in gallon containers with lovely artwork gracing the beautiful blue bottle. Pure rose water it was, bottled only yards from where the flowers grew on a sunny hillside near the Mediterranean, overlooking the perfumed town of Grasse in southern France. Or bottles of orange water, made from millions of fragile white blossoms with their splash of orange center, ranged the length of a pharmacy shelf.

One bath that must have been heavenly was the gelatin bath. It required 500 grams of gelatin mixed in four quarts of warm water. This was then added to your tub and it was filled with water. Today, that bath would be prohibitive in cost.

An earlier generation of Japanese women prized smoothly polished skin which resembled fine porcelain, according to a woman from that country who continues this fine tradition of her grandmother. Brown rice polish is tucked into a small bag, only large enough to fit comfortably into the hand; with this, you scour your entire body while sitting in a tub of warm water.

Yo, who came as a war bride to this country, remembers comments from her mother and grandmother on the use of this beauty grain. Whenever Japanese women with beautiful skin would appear, invariably, Yo recalls references to rice polish as the chief factor in their excellent skin textures.

So, find a mail-order house supplying rice polish, which is simply the inner bran layers from brown rice, removed during the refining process. Or check into a health food store, and buy a pound of this lovely powder. Make a small drawstring bag, fill it with the rice polish, and use it as a washcloth for the entire body. Change the polish after every two baths, at least.

REMOVING SKIN DISCOLORATION

Nowadays the majority of skin splotching seems to come from the use of birth control pills. To their great alarm, women have found that though this "pregnancy mask" sometimes disappears upon cessation of use of The Pill, too frequently a brownish shadow remains.

This is a modern complaint, and there are as yet no reports on the effects of home remedies on these discolorations. But in earlier days women suffered the same affliction during pregnancy, and coped with it by using various washes aimed at bleaching away the shadowy tinge. Many times this "moth patch," as it was quaintly called, disappeared by itself. But women are always eager to assist the removal of an unattractive stigma, so the following remedies were devised. You might try them, one at a time, if you're faced with modern moth patches.

But remember, in earlier days even as today, these discolorations stemmed, in some instances, from true pregnancies instead of today's induced semblance. For the hormones and estrogens which make The Pill effective act to produce a continual false pregnancy and, in that sense, if you are a Pill user, your body believes it is in a continual state of pregnancy.

Since all of the remedies listed are of fruit and vegetable origin, they should not be harmful unless you are allergic to a specific fruit or vegetable. If the skin stings uncomfortably, remove the solution and rinse thoroughly.

Since this is the month the bogs are producing their harvest, you might want to use a fresh cranberry lotion. Crammed with vitamin C and a good bleaching agent when used externally, cranberries should also be eaten at the same time they are used on the moth patches. For best results, do not oversweeten or overcook them and use only honey for sweetening.

You may try the berries as a bleaching agent by using the freshly squeezed juice, or by heating a handful of berries until the juice runs out and using that.

Pat into the discolored skin area and allow the liquid to dry on the skin. Rinse in warm, then cool, water and pat dry. Apply a film of vegetable or nut oil to avoid skin irritation. One treatment alone won't do much, but keep a close check on your skin to avoid irritation.

Yogurt is also an excellent means of producing more even skin tone. Use plain, of course, patting across the discolored area. Allow it to dry, and rinse it away. Or try buttermilk for similar results. Or stewed, unsweetened dried apricots, reduced to a pulpy smoothness in a blender. Apply to the discolored area and lie on a slantboard for 30 minutes.

With any of these skin bleaches, rinse away and then pat in a film of oil to prevent possible irritation.

APPLE CREAM FOR FRESHENING
SKIN TONE

A wealth of nutrition and natural cosmetics are still lying in the garden, stacked up at roadside stands and flooding the markets in October. As though in one generous fling, nature wants to go out in glory. And so she shall. Mounds of brilliant orange pumpkins, sheaves of golden corn, and baskets of apples so crisp the skins seem near to bursting are waiting to appear on the table and to be used cosmetically.

Apples anyone? Eat them and use them on your face for a refreshing and moisturizing lotion. In the diet, they bring vitamins B, C, and G, in addition to minerals. Acting as a demulcent, they cleanse the teeth. A study made at Michigan State University over a three-year period indicated students who ate two apples a day were more relaxed, had fewer headaches, and experienced less emotional distress than those who ate no apples. In addition, apple eaters have fewer skin diseases. So Eve knew what she was doing, after all. She may have disappointed God, but look what she did for humanity.

Externally, an apple facial will feed, cleanse, tighten, and soften the skin. Though any fruit can be beneficial if it is applied directly to the skin, adding apples to a cream base gives you super benefits by including protein from egg, potassium from apple cider vinegar, and vitamin E from cold pressed oil.

Apple Cream Facial

1 teaspoon lemon juice	2 tablespoons beauty cream
½ peeled and chopped apple	base (see below)
2 teaspoons honey	

Mix lemon juice over the chopped apple and put all ingredients into the blender. Blend at slow, then high, speed until smooth. Massage gently into face and neck area and leave on for 20 minutes. Rinse away with warm water, without using soap. Blot dry.

Beauty Cream Base

2 egg yolks

2 tablespoons apple cider
vinegar

¾ cup safflower oil

Put the egg yolks, vinegar, and ¼ cup oil into blender and beat on highest speed. As the mixture thickens, slowly pour in the remaining oil in a slow steady stream and continue to beat until it is fully emulsified. Use alone as a facial or as a base to which other beauty foods are added.

VIRGIN'S MILK

From the earliest days of exposure to the sun or dust from chariot wheels or working over a fire which cooked dinner but also clogged their skin with soot, women have searched for really effective pore cleansers.

Preference has always been given to astringent lotions or preparations which cleanse, contract, and tighten the skin. There is a feeling of new and pulsing life on the face when you use a prepared water or lotion which, in contracting the skin, brings a swifter blood flow and cleanses under tissue while removing debris from the surface.

Virgin's milk is an ancient and valued lotion which does double duty in cleansing and softening a slack complexion. The simple ingredients are among the most effective means to restore a neglected complexion.

For this much-lauded face wash, pour ¼ cup of rose water into a bottle. Add, one drop at a time, four drops of tincture of benzoin, shaking vigorously after each addition. Apply the solution with a cotton ball to a freshly scrubbed face.

CHESTNUT PASTE FOR THE HANDS

The first chestnuts are in the markets, and if you have chestnut trees, you are vying with the busy squirrels who realize the great nutritional value of this mineral-rich food, which contains both sulfur and manganese. Sulfur is a vital element in the hair cell and is essential for good hair growth. The value of manganese lies in its role as an enzyme activator.

Chestnuts seem to be more highly valued in Europe than in North America. Perhaps we lost touch with this nut food following the deadly blight of the American chestnut trees a generation or so ago, when the disease swept across the country. But zealous growers and lovers of this satisfying food have replaced the weaker American tree with a tree combining different qualities, and now there is a resurgence of these nuts on the market.

Aside from the delicious wisdom of buying freshly roasted chestnuts from street vendors all over Europe to eat with the fingers or to serve at table as a vegetable or dessert, Europeans use them in various cosmetics. The hand cream described here is an ancient formula used in remote regions of Italy, where practices hundreds of years old have continued without interruption to this day.

I came across this recipe for chestnut paste for the hands in Orvieto, one of the magnificent hilltowns near Florence. No one in town knew its age. It had always been used, the innkeeper's wife insisted. Why she remembered her grandmother pounding the mealy nuts into a fine powder and mixing them with sweet olive oil, amber honey, and the yolk of an egg.

Recipe? Who needed a recipe? Everyone knew how to prepare chestnut paste for the hands. Just a bit of this and that and a few chestnuts.

But substituting chestnuts in a formula for almond paste, I think I have come up with a good hand paste that is different, beneficial, and fun to prepare.

Chestnut Hand Paste

¼ cup honey
¼ cup finely ground chestnut meal

2 teaspoons egg yolk
¼ cup sweet almond oil

Heat the honey over hot water in a dish large enough to allow for thorough mixing and kneading. Add the meal and dissolve by thorough beating. Add the egg yolk and beat it in. Very slowly add the almond oil, a bit at a time, and knead the mixture until a paste is formed. Adjust the egg yolk if more malleability is needed. Rub into the hands and hold briefly under warm water. Blot nearly dry and wring the hands to massage in the remaining paste.

YOGURT AND BREWER'S YEAST FACIAL

The elusive quality of truly glowing skin is eagerly sought by women who usually think they can achieve it from a tube or jar. The store-bought cream must subsequently be scoured from the face to prevent clogging. This method cannot be favorably compared with the bloom that grows from within and lights the complexion with a faint flush of health rather than a dab of flat color.

You can grow your own color with a stimulating brewer's yeast and yogurt mask. It is an excellent idea to take the yeast internally as well as apply it as a facial covering to bring penetrating stimulation. This beauty food can put a luster in your hair, life in your skin, and energy in your walk. There are many concentrated beauty foods available, but yeast just about heads the list with all its attributes.

It is a no-nonsense food. Tastes dreadful, but if you will suffer its taste, it will repay you in a thousand healthy, beautiful ways. And you can disguise its taste in a glass of tomato juice, holding your breath as it goes down. Before or after each meal, mix 1 teaspoon of yeast in a glass of liquid. Gradually increase the amount to 1 tablespoon, over a period of time, until you are taking 3 tablespoons of the yeast in liquid every day.

When you see what this beauty food will do for skin, hair, and nails, it will become dearer to you than a chocolate eclair. And do a lot more for you.

One word of caution here. While brewer's yeast does indeed offer a wealth of B vitamins and certainly will enhance anyone's daily diet, it would be a wise idea to increase your intake of calcium at the same time. The reason for this is that brewer's yeast contains a great deal of phosphorus but very little calcium. When phosphorus intake is higher than calcium intake, the latter is removed from the body by the action of the former.

To ensure a proper balance, then, increase your calcium intake, along with vitamin D for proper assimilation of the calcium. The calcium increase can come from milk or yogurt, or from calcium tablets. The synergistic action of the various vitamins and minerals shows the mosaic of nutrition and reminds us that we should examine our diets carefully to be sure we are getting all the nutrients our bodies require.

When you cover your face with this wonder, B-complex food

mask, there is a delicious stimulation as the yeast, in drying, contracts and draws faster coursing blood just beneath the skin to feed and cleanse it. You get the best results if the mask dries on your face while you are upended on the slantboard. This requires 15 to 30 minutes to be fully effective. And the mask should be completely dry before you remove it. If you've put on a thick covering, it could take even longer, but a thin to moderate covering is ample.

You can enrich even further the wealth of B vitamins in brewer's yeast by adding yogurt to it. There is a predigested protein feast in the yogurt used to create a soft paste when combined with yeast. With its contribution of vitamin B and its protein and surface skin cleansing qualities, yogurt helps make this a million-dollar mask for dull skin.

Stir 2 teaspoons of yogurt (unsweetened, unembellished, and, if possible, made from raw milk) into a teaspoon of dried brewer's yeast. If needed, add additional yogurt to make a soft, easily spreadable paste. Pat onto the face and neck areas. Leave on until completely dry. A face cloth dipped in warm water softens and helps remove the hardened mask. Rinse thoroughly and rub a thin layer of salad oil into the undereye area.

BRAN HAIR WASH

Why does the caterpillar seem to grow a more fuzzy body covering some years? Old almanacs say this is in anticipation of a long cold winter. And the bear and possum are now sleek and heavy-haired as they get ready to tuck themselves away for a winter's nap. With October here, it is indeed time to think of digging in for the winter. But while the hibernating creatures of the world seem to grow thick masses of fur with no effort, we must look to our own resources for fuller hair growth.

Why was hair once so abundant, so richly endowed with length and strength? Have you ever seen an old portrait or photograph of a person with skimpy locks? Women always seemed to have had masses of thick hair wound around their heads, braided into ropes, or massed atop their heads and anchored with massive tortoiseshell combs. Those combs alone would attest to superior hair. Few women today have the thickness of hair to hold those lavish adornments you find only in antique shows now.

What happened? Could it be our detergent shampoo, our diets, or a combination of both? If you seriously want to improve your hair and help it to grow and become easier to manage and a thing of beauty, then be prepared to work for it. There is no product on the market that can be slathered on the head and do what natural, unprocessed, and living food will do.

In addition to upgrading your diet to eliminate all processed foods, you will want to use a shampoo which nourishes and cleans at the same time. Perhaps one solution to disappearing hair beauty lies in the use of this treatment, an old German formula which was popular when women spent an extra hour just winding their hair around their heads to get it out of the way.

Pour 1 cup of bran (not the fine type, but the whole bran itself) into 4 cups of cold water. Bring it slowly to a boil and simmer for 5 minutes. Strain through gauze and add a capful of herbal shampoo. Massage thoroughly into the hair and rinse out. Now, beat 2 egg yolks into a cup of warm water and massage this into both scalp and hair, lingering over the job to coat every strand and guarantee saturation. Rinse out with tepid water and dry the hair with additional massage, toweling for stimulation.

Try this shampoo weekly and see whether your locks don't improve considerably. And you might want to scout out one of those exquisite tortoiseshell combs for future use.

APHRODISIAC FOR OCTOBER

Since temptation began in the garden with an apple, it might be wise to recognize the most potent fruit of them all as an aphrodisiac. Aside from the apple's vitamin A, B, and C content, there are also sulfur and magnesium to get the glands going. The apple's tranquilizing effects also leave the body more receptive to stimulating influences.

It might be a good idea to produce a provocative apple dish just to see whether it is as effective as the sorcerer's book says. And if it doesn't bring results in that department, relax and enjoy the knowledge that the apple is really great for the teeth and that, in consequence, all is not lost.

Applesauce in the Raw

6 apples, peeled, cored, and   ¼ cup fresh orange juice
    chopped   honey
1 slice lemon

Blend one-half of the apples and remaining ingredients in the blender until ground. Add the other three apples and blend smooth. Beat in honey to taste.

BEAUTY BREATHING

October's air is fresh and brisk, so now is the time to learn good breathing, which is also beauty breathing. A vital component of beauty is sufficient oxygen. Not only is this commodity life-giving, but it is life-sustaining and improving, and then some. Many people have found a supposed secret to vitality and beauty through correct breathing exercises which bring additional oxygen to the body. In this manner, the increased oxygen purifies and cleans the blood more thoroughly and the entire body profits from the fresh blood supply that will revitalize and feed even far-away hair roots, the last place on the body to receive nourishment.

Deep breathing can flush the body with oxygen at moments of strain or stress, reducing the impact of a traumatic experience. Usually, when a person is under strain or feeling tense, she has a tendency to breathe shallowly, further stunting the body's oxygen supply just when it is most needed. Practice will teach that, on the contrary, a deeply indrawn breath will take the edge off the worst disaster and allow the mind to retain its decisionmaking abilities in comparative calm. This is because the mental functions aren't shortchanged on life-giving oxygen.

The importance of deep breathing cannot be overemphasized. The entire appearance and general condition of your body is dependent on the good functioning of the inner organs. By increasing your circulation, you can not only better maintain your body but can help keep excess weight down through an improved metabolism.

By deep breathing, the abdominal muscles are given extra exercise which aids in digestion and food assimilation. Go for a walk after a meal, and do some deep beauty breathing exercises. In this way you can assist the metabolism to convert food into energy rather than permit it to become excess flesh on the body. When done correctly and frequently enough, diaphragmatic, or deep, breathing, prevents oxygen starvation and wards off premature aging. Try to get into the habit of beauty breathing. There are other names for it, but I call it beauty breathing here to remind you of its great benefits in that area.

The general tone of your life will improve when you include this among other good health practices in your program of physical improvement. All of these attentions to the body are parts of a greater whole. There is little reason to believe that one tiny act of charity toward the body will be effective or change things drastically. But treated as a whole, though approached in several directions, the body will respond and grow in health and beauty.

Just as important as deep breathing is the expelling of impurities from the lungs afterward. It isn't enough to inhale deeply, for in providing the oxygen to cleanse the bloodstream of wastes and toxins, you must also provide a means to dispose of these wastes. Exhaling just as intently as you inhale creates a balanced breathing which leaves the body refreshed, alert, and vigorous.

To do this correctly, gently push the air from the top of the chest first, then the middle area, and finally the abdomen, which flattens as the last stale air is forced from the lungs.

When you begin deep beauty breathing, remember it should not replace the regular chest breathing you normally do, except at specific times. It should be practiced only during moments of strain or distress and during exercises when the body has a greater need for increased oxygen. A refreshing midmorning or afternoon break is as simple as finding an open window or door, or merely stepping outside and drawing in several long, slow, deep beauty breaths. Take the same length of time to expel the used air from the body. Contrary to deep beauty in-breathing, exhaling is done by slowly releasing the air from the mouth, with some assistance from the abdominal muscles in expelling all the stale air.

Though beauty breathing can be performed walking, standing, seated, or lying down, it is advantageous to try it first while lying on the floor. In this manner, you can monitor the process and correct any tendency to shallow breathe because it is easier to check with the body in this position.

From your position on the floor, with your arms by your sides, relax your entire body. Very slowly breathe through the nostrils with the mouth closed, and send the indrawn oxygen to the lowest part of the lungs. Place your hand lightly on your abdomen, and you will feel it rise as air is pushed downward. The chest and shoulders must not move, and only the rib cage and abdomen should expand.

With the full expansion of the lungs, very slowly release your breath, draining your body of the used air, or carbon dioxide, first from the upper portion of the lungs, then the middle section, and finally the lower region. It is this area, the lower region, that is seldom completely emptied, and it is here, then, that toxic wastes remain. To prevent that, consciously push out the last remaining air.

Repeat the deep beauty breathing two or three times, but no more than that in the beginning, as an overdose of unaccustomed oxygen can lead to hyperventilation, creating dizziness. After a week or two, you can increase the depth breathing, but do not be extravagant in its practice at any one time. Rather, space your beauty breathing throughout the day, two or three deep breaths at a time. And always try to deep breathe when you are in fresh air rather than a polluted, or overbreathed, atmosphere. Also use deep breathing when exercising or under stress.

BREAKFASTS FOR OCTOBER

⌘

Baked apples
Potato pancakes*
Herbal tea

Cranberry juice
Cornmeal mush cooked with dates
Herbal tea

Baked pears
Date nut bread with eggs
Herbal tea

Tangerine wedges
Molasses and millet cereal (recipe on p. 45)
Herbal tea

Bananas and cream
Eggs served on toasted potato slices*
Herbal tea

Fresh orange slices
Apple pancakes (recipe on p. 165)
Herbal tea

Cranberry juice
Sprout omelet
Herbal tea

LUNCHES FOR OCTOBER

❦

Broth with brown rice
Avocado and banana salad
Yogurt

Bean soup
Apple and cheese bowl
Yogurt

Apple soup*
Sprout salad (recipe on p. 47)
Corn sticks
Yogurt

String bean and onion salad
Mushroom chop suey
Yogurt

Mushroom soup
Whole grain sandwiches
Yogurt

Cabbage soup
Cornmeal chapaties (recipe on p. 83)
Yogurt

Onion soup (recipe on p. 94)
Toasted whole grain cheese sandwiches
Yogurt

DINNERS FOR OCTOBER

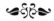

Tongue with raisins
Potatoes in skins
Brussels sprouts

Broiled brains
Steamed mung sprouts
Buckwheat groats with oil and lemon juice

Vegetable omelet*
Savory garbanzos
Steamed Chinese cabbage with lemon oil dressing

Baked fish with tomato sauce
Winter squash
Broccoli

Stuffed mushrooms
Brown rice with parsley
Steamed cabbage and green peppers

Sautéed liver dipped in wheat germ
Parsnips
Broiled green peppers

Sautéed kidneys
Stewed apple slices
Corn

RECIPES FOR OCTOBER

Potato Pancakes

3 grated potatoes
sea salt to taste
½ cup minced onion

1 beaten egg
1 tablespoon vegetable oil

Grate the potatoes and mix in salt, onion, and egg. Drop from a tablespoon into an oiled and heated skillet. Cook to a crispy brown on both sides.

Toasted Potato Slices

Slice scrubbed Idaho potatoes fairly thin and dip in salad oil. Place on cookie sheet and bake in 450 degree oven until golden brown. Use as bread.

Apple Soup

1 cup chicken broth
1 cup milk
½ cup grated Swiss cheese or
  any natural unprocessed
  cheese

1 teaspoon curry powder
2 chopped apples

Simmer all ingredients together for 5 minutes. Place in blender until liquefied. Serve hot with a tablespoon of grated cheese on top.

Vegetable Omelet

1 minced carrot
2 minced stalks of celery
1 minced green pepper
1 minced onion
6 eggs

½ cup milk
seasoning
2 tablespoons oil
minced parsley

Sauté vegetables in oil until tender. Pour eggs beaten with milk and seasoning over the vegetables; cover and simmer until the omelet puffs up. Turn over and cook until slightly firm. Sprinkle with parsley. Serves four.

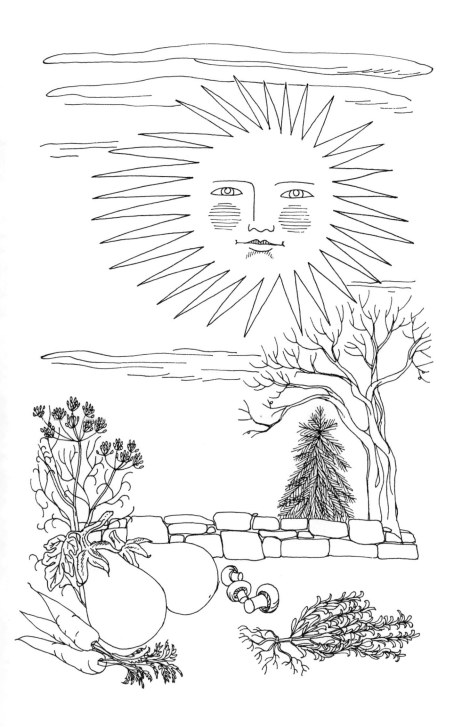

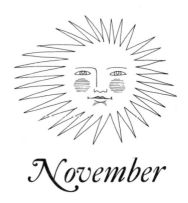

November

The wild November comes at last
Beneath a veil of rain;
The latest of her race, she takes
The Autumn's vacant throne;
She has but one short moon to live,
And she must live alone.

R. H. Stoddard: "November"

Called practically and unromantically Slaughter Month in earlier times, in reference to the preparation of food for the winter months, this Wind Month and Fog Month seems to leave everyone despondent in its appearance.

No sun—no moon!
No morn—no noon
No dawn—no dusk—no proper time of day.
No warmth, no cheerfulness, no healthful ease,
No comfortable feel in any member—
No shade, no shine, no butterflies, no bees.
No fruits, no flowers, no leaves, no birds!—
November!

Thomas Hood

And yet, this dreaded month is not all bad. There are things to do and prepare from which more agreeable months would lure you away. This is the time to build up your body, to make exotic and homey preparations, and to examine the needs of your body and cater to it.

Whether from the cold winds sweeping out of the north, or the drying desert sun, this is the month to protect the winter body; to lavish extra care and attention on it, and to replenish, restore, and guard the body's own protective mantle.

Sometimes we are thrust rather brutally from the lovely golden days of autumn into the harshest of sudden winter storms, and there is always disbelief that winter came so early this year. Suddenly all the warmth absorbed from the summer sun, and all the soft breezes and abundance from nature's garden seem taken away. Only grayness and cold are left. But we adjust. And look forward to December. First, though, November must be gotten through. It will be, and can be, more enjoyably endured if a person knows she looks great, feels well, and is in top condition and can ride out the storm of winter.

There are many ways to do this. A good diet, exercises, and loving body care—they are all a form of insurance and pay handsome dividends in a more attractive appearance and sense of well-being.

YUCATAN SKIN SMOOTHER

Something exotic is needed this cold, damp month, in order to spur a better blood flow, create a warm glow in the skin, and to enable one to turn one's back on November and its chill. A south-of-the-border formula should do it. In the sparsely settled areas of Yucatan, a traveler comes across remote villages where women have incredibly fine skin. Pores are so small and refined they seem nonexistent. And the texture of all the body skin is honey smooth in appearance.

Fruits and vegetables figure heavily in the diet here, but there is more. These dark-eyed women use materials at hand and produce a facial pack which is allowed to dry on the skin, then is carefully removed with warm water, after which an oil is gently rubbed into the skin.

The formula, as given me, was incomplete, for my Yucatan informant could not tell me how the third ingredient, a root grown only near Yucatan, could possibly be purchased north of the border. But we arrived at a good substitute, and here we have essentially the same simple skin smoother.

Mix together 2 tablespoons of lime juice and 2 tablespoons of raw honey. Blend in 3 tablespoons of rice polish or rice flour. Spread the paste across the face and neck areas and allow to dry completely, around 30 minutes. Carefully rub away with a wet washcloth. Oil lightly but thoroughly by rubbing gently upward into the skin with a salad oil.

BALSAM FOR THE HANDS

The Indians had a basic approach to the winter season. Fresh bear's grease was carefully massaged into the body, and teas of dried elder bark were drunk to increase circulation. In this manner, they were safe from chafing skin; dry, peeling, and flaky tissue, and warm at the same time, considering all the air that must have crept under those uninsulated blankets.

But what an aching time for sensitive hands. And no amount of bear's grease or innocuous liquid poured from a pretty bottle and labeled hand lotion seems to benefit delicate hand tissue which dries to an uncomfortable state during this month unless extra care is provided.

Honey is one of the most lavish and simple skin protectors known. Its lubricating, nourishing, and velvety qualities pamper roughened skin texture and, used daily, it can help overcome reddened, overworked, and dry skin. Add a smidgen of benzoin to that and you've increased the benefits. This balsamic resin from trees growing in Sumatra and Java is used in the finest skin preparations. So feel pampered as you make your own paste. Add wax from the honeycomb and you've further protected your hands from raw, windy onslaughts when you forget your gloves, or even when you are working indoors. While this is a hand cleanser more than a conditioner, it is softening at the same time, and offers a wealth of protection. Be patient with the time-consuming task of preparation. It was impatience with the old methods that brought about the present chemical age which, though it has its place in a technical world, somehow seems out of place in preparations which come in contact with the body.

Honey Balsam Paste for Hand Cleansing

40 grams of pure castile soap	10 grams of tincture of benzoin
50 grams of honey	30 grams of white beeswax

Shave the castile soap into thin strips and melt with the honey in the top of a double boiler. Blend together and then beat the benzoin into the mixture thoroughly before adding the wax. Beat together and when completely blended, remove from the heat and put into a container. Use this paste for the hands instead of soap. Dip into the container for a dollop, wet the hands, and massage the paste in by holding the hands under a slowly running warm water faucet. Blot dry.

FENNEL FACIAL

The legend has persisted down through the ages that the herb fennel will remove fine facial lines if used often enough. Why doubt it now? Reach back for earlier practices and profit, for using nature to aid life is only wise and practical. Besides, this aromatic herb with its bits of golden flower heads and feathery leaves is an attractive garden plant.

Aside from firming aging skin tissue, fennel can be brewed into tea which, drunk daily, is considered an aid in fighting obesity. In whatever way it is used, fennel is a beauty plant and should be in every garden, or on every herb shelf, and used often.

Fennel Facial to Remove Lines

Make a strong tea by adding 1 tablespoon of fennel seed to 1 cup of boiling water. Steep covered until cool. Mix 1 teaspoon of the fennel liquid with 1 teaspoon of raw honey. Stir in 2 tablespoons of yogurt and mix together. Apply to the face and leave for 30 minutes, or until it is completely dry. Wash away with warm water, then cool, and blot dry.

For everyday facial cleansing, make a tea of 1 tablespoon of fennel seed steeped in 1 cup of boiling water. Keep refrigerated until needed. Dip cotton pads into the liquid to remove makeup, and you've an excellent skin cleanser with strengthening qualities. Do not use soap or additional water, but rather, blot the skin dry with tissues. This wash leaves a fresh, clean fragrance.

UNDEREYE AREA

Problems of the undereye area seem to affect women of all ages, and as winter approaches, the shadows always seem more prominent. Even women in their twenties complain of dark circles and shadowy tinges. Dry, sagging skin increases the look of age, and the problem should be worked on daily.

There is always the possibility of systemic cause which can quickly reflect itself in various eye conditions. Difficulties with the kidneys can result in puffiness under the eyes. Vitamin deficiencies through faulty nutrition or assimilation will quickly manifest themselves in unattractive undereye skin conditions. After checking to correct and eliminate these disorders, there are external applications which can help restore elasticity and life to the undereye tissue.

Use the restorative slantboard to get double beauty mileage. Lie down on the board and place a warm, not hot, tea bag on each eye. Be sure to cover the entire undereye area with the bag. This is helpful in softening lines and resting the eyes themselves.

Witch hazel pads can also be refreshing and restore a sparkle to the eyes if kept on for twenty to thirty minutes. Dip cotton pads into this herbal liquid and apply on the lids while lying down with your eyes closed.

Always oil the undereye area after using the moistened pads. A thin film of sesame seed oil is excellent, but any vegetable, nut, or seed oil will do.

To tighten this problem area, beat together one teaspoon of honey and one teaspoon of unbeaten egg white. Gently pat this into the skin and allow it to dry. Rinse away in warm water. Never rub anything in this area, for the thin, almost oilless skin under the eye is extremely fragile, and heavy massaging can do irreparable harm.

SKIN TISSUE CREAM

As the weather grows raw, it's a good idea to let the skin nourish itself from an overnight application of a food with special nutritive qualities. This is a painless way of building up the skin. Don't wait until the aging process commences before following daily or nightly beauty schedules for body maintenance, for then it is much more difficult. Rather, start early in life with simple, easy-to-put-together skin foods and don't miss a day using them.

Lanolin is the fat most closely resembling that in the human body and is thus all the more readily absorbed by the skin. Add to this good base the splendid effects of sweet almond oil and you have a tissue cream which can soften the most difficult and neglected of skins.

Melt together in a glass custard cup 4 tablespoons of lanolin (U.S.P., hydrous) and 3 tablespoons of sweet almond oil. Beat together as it melts and slowly add 2 tablespoons of mineral water. Add a few drops of perfume, if you wish, though it is always better to avoid the sometimes irritating perfumes in skin preparations. Pour the thoroughly blended mixture into a jar and use nightly or daily.

PINE BATH

Many of the fashionable spas in Germany offer an unusual bath to their guests which relaxes both nerves and muscles, soaks away aches, and produces a tonic effect on the body. A concentrate of the balsamic resin from pine needles is added to a tub of water, and you soak in this comforting brew until your body feels free of various discomforts. A true winter scent—and no unpleasant effects. A good cleansing agent, the pine extract also stimulates the circulation and produces an invigorated and restored, yet calm and rested body and mind.

The extract used in the spas is available in this country now, but be sure to get the true pine extract, not a synthetic pine-scented preparation. Read the label to be sure you are getting the real thing.

If you would like to experiment on your own, and you have a pine tree or so, gather 1 quart of the green needles and drop them into 2 quarts of briskly boiling water. Simmer gently for 5 or 6 minutes. Strain the water into a tub half filled with warm water and plan to spend at least 20 minutes soaking in this. Do not use soap in this bath, but rather, depend on a vigorous toweling to complete the soothing and cleansing action of the resinous pine needles.

BANANA FACIAL

A banana mask can bring relief to a tautened, dry winter skin by feeding it with vitamins A, B, C, and G, plus calcium, iron, and phosphorus. In addition, rub the inner side of the banana peel across dry, ailing hands before disposing of it. The invaluable oils in the banana skin can do a splendid softening and even healing job on distressed hands.

Mash enough completely ripe banana to give you 2 tablespoons of pulp. Beat in ½ teaspoon of cream and gently rub this into an herb- or milk-washed face. Leave on for 30 minutes before rinsing away with warm, then cool, water.

COLD WEATHER CREAM

A lubricating and emollient type of cream is good protection against chafed skin during winter. By applying a thin film of this cream nightly or daily, you can help avoid the unattractive, flaking skin that can accompany cold weather.

Cocoa butter from the roasted cocoa bean is considered one of the most natural of body applications because of its tendency to be absorbed by the skin and leave it comparatively greaseless. As such, it is the basis for many salves and ointments and it is used beneficially in cosmetic creams because it melts at body temperature. When you combine it with lanolin and a cold pressed oil, you create a triple-rich protective, nourishing, and smoothing cream which should prove priceless to your winter collection of cosmetics.

Melt over hot water 2 tablespoons of lanolin and blend in 2 tablespoons of cocoa butter, 2 tablespoons of mineral water, and 6 tablespoons of wheat germ oil. Beat together thoroughly and pour into a lidded jar. Apply to skin which has been freshly scrubbed and then rinsed with a few drops of apple cider vinegar in the water. Blot dry and immediately rub in a small quantity of the cream by using upward, circular movements.

SKIN FOOD LOTION

Those interested in early beauty preparations and methods to preserve a fresh and dewy complexion, again and again run across one standby formula that seems to have served generations of women admirably, and that no woman questioned. It obviously stands on its own merit, for the formula was passed along from mother to daughter, and so today, thanks to those past generations of women, we have a superb and simple concoction which does indeed work. If used over a period of time, oatmeal skin lotion brings a softness and suppleness to even tired and neglected complexions. Remember, not just a splash and a promise to do better later; this is a daily, or twice daily, lotion.

Oatmeal Skin Food Lotion

Boil 1 cup of steel-cut oatmeal in 1 pint of boiling water until a clear liquid forms. Use a double boiler for this to prevent sticking, for this oatmeal is not the usual instant type, but the grainy, unprocessed kind. Strain the clear liquid through gauze, boil the oatmeal another 5 minutes, and strain again. When the liquid cools, add enough rose water or orange flower water to create a milklike consistency. Keep refrigerated. Be sure the rose water or orange flower water is pure and does not contain any alcohol. Usually you can purchase this in a gourmet shop; its place of origin is France.

TO THICKEN THE HAIR

The coat of the caterpillar becomes deep pile in November, and the birds nestle snugly beneath layers of down and feathers, all figured out according to each's winter needs. Fine. But what about your hair? Shouldn't that take on an added fullness to give warmth against a winter wind? Nature seldom if ever errs, so why aren't we prepared for colder months with a rewardingly thick head of hair?

Perhaps because we are given the means to help ourselves, it is left to us to put together concoctions which nourish and stimulate good hair growth. Besides, there has to be some compensation for being a caterpillar.

An old and favored recipe for thickening the hair comes down through household journals and doesn't seem to vary much in its ingredients—or in praises for effectiveness. It is a bother to prepare because of the distilling apparatus required. If you have this piece of equipment and care to brew your own, you may be able to influence hair growth.

Recipe for Thickening the Hair

| 1 handful rosemary flowers | 1 quart white wine |
| 1/2 pound of raw honey | 1/4 pint of sweet almond oil |

Mix rosemary and honey with the wine, distill them together. Add the sweet almond oil and shake well. When using, pour a little into a cup, warm it, and rub into the roots of the hair.

If this seems too much bother, use plain rosemary tea rubbed into the roots. This appears never to fail.

EGG WASH FOR DIFFICULT HAIR

In winter, all problems look worse. Hair ends are split, the locks themselves flyaway, and the lifeless condition seems beyond any redemption. Now is the time for the straight egg treatment. Pure egg yolk can be the answer to a multitude of hair problems, most having to do with lack of nutrition getting through to the roots in order to nourish them and stimulate growth.

No other shampoo should be used with egg wash. The egg itself not only feeds, but also cleanses better than any shampoo known. At the same time, it does not remove any vital hair oils.

Apple cider vinegar is mixed with the egg yolk to increase assimilation of the protein by the hair strands. There are those who will argue that the egg cannot be absorbed by the hair, but that is nonsense, for all you have to do is try this marvelous formula for resurrecting tormented hair, and you've proof right there that the egg and vinegar combination is truly one of the greats in hair care.

Egg Wash

Mix 1 teaspoon of apple cider vinegar with 1 cup of warm water. Beat 2 egg yolks into the liquid and carefully massage this into both hair and scalp. Spend several minutes working the mixture into all areas of both scalp and hair. Now tie a plastic bag around your hair and secure it to increase scalp heat within the bag and quicken assimilation by the hair shafts.

Allow the bag to remain for at least 5 minutes before removing. Pour ¼ cup warm water or just enough to create a nice lather through the hair and vigorously work the resultant lather throughout the hair. Rinse with a spray attachment under warm water. Continue rinsing and massaging until the water runs clear, which takes longer than a regular shampoo. Pour 1 tablespoon of apple cider vinegar into a quart of warm water and use this for the last rinse. Towel dry the hair.

VENUS CREAM FOR CHAPPED FACE

Sometimes, in spite of careful applications of a soothing cream, oil, or other emollient, the denuding winds of winter can chap the facial tissues and produce an uncomfortable and unsightly mottling with stinging red patches. When this happens, a protective covering can be put to excellent use to prevent further damage and permit the rich mixture of oils and creams to heal the sensitive area.

Venus cream came first from Paris at least 100 years ago. Its softening and protective qualities made it a favorite there and here. But you almost never hear of it now outside old journals and cosmetic books. In general, I am opposed to the use of wax on the face because it is a non-nutritive substance, but to combat chapped winter skin, I would stretch a point and prepare a jar of Venus cream. When the facial tissue clears up, a good steaming and oiling could then remove any trace of the wax, since only a small amount is used in the formula.

Venus Cream

¼ ounce spermaceti
¼ ounce white beeswax
4 ounces sweet almond oil
4 ounces cocoa butter

2 ounces lanolin
1 teaspoon Balsam of Peru
2 teaspoons orange flower
   water

Melt the first five ingredients together and stir in the Balsam of Peru. Remove from the heat and allow the mixture to settle before pouring off the clear portion and adding the orange water to it. Dispose of the sediment. Stir briskly, while the cream is still warm, until it hardens.

Apply Venus cream after exposure to harsh weather. Leave on one hour and remove by bathing the face in warm water and blotting it gently dry. These ingredients are all soothing to weather-distressed skin. The balsam has long been popular in the Far East, where it is used in flavoring drinks and as a scenting medium and fixative agent for sachets and potpourris. Its penetrating scent makes it a pleasant addition to ointments and creams.

PASTILLES FOR BURNING

Add cheer to November by beating up a batch of old-fashioned pastilles to burn. A summertime project in the days when people gathered their scents fresh from garden, woods, and field, making pastilles, or incense, can be a pleasant November occupation if you use botanical supplies. While away a day preparing them and then enchant a long evening.

Originally used to disguise strong odors, pastilles achieved a certain elegance during the reign of George III by being placed in silver containers made especially for them. They were whisked into the dining halls along with the dessert to overcome the heavier odors of strong foods. From the halls of the palace, they found their way, in more modest containers, into cottages and have since been appreciated no matter where they burn.

Pastilles

1½ teaspoons potassium nitrate
6 oz powdered charcoal
4 teaspoons gum benzoin
2 teaspoons frankincense
2 teaspoons storax

8 teaspoons cascarilla bark
2 teaspoons yellow sandalwood
2 teaspoons gum tragacanth
water

Reduce all solids to a powder. Dissolve the gum tragacanth in enough water to produce a mucilage which will be moist enough to blend all the ingredients together in a soft mass. Form this soft material into small cones and dry in a very low oven or on some warm surface. To use, place on any hot surface, or set the tip of a cone on fire, extinguish the blaze, and allow the pastille to smolder in order to release its perfume.

The ingredients required for these pastilles are all available from a botanical supply house.

APHRODISIAC FOR NOVEMBER

Some very unromantic items are indirectly associated with love. Glands, depending on their condition, can often determine your interest and whether you are interesting. A sluggish disposition never produced an exciting person, nor does a prematurely aged woman or man have great enthusiasm for the various joys of living.

Hormone production determines the degree of activity of the glands. And since hormones are composed mostly of protein, it is vital to have an adequate amount of this nutrient in the diet.

Along with other important minerals, iodine plays an important role in stimulating the body. For a really smashing evening, you might want to try oysters broiled with sea kelp, or dulse, for seasoning. This may sound far from romantic, but it is a powerful meal, because the iodine content in this dish is as high as you can get. In fact, around the turn of the century, a product made from wild Portuguese oysters became almost a mania because of its aphrodisiacal qualities. And its potency was easily traced to its high mineral content.

EXERCISES FOR BUST DEVELOPMENT

Since the breasts are essentially glandular, they cannot in themselves be changed noticeably in growth by exercises. Rather, one must approach problem breasts by concentrating on the pectoral muscles in the chest that provide support for the breasts, through connecting tissues of the glands of the chest.

By strengthening the pectoral muscles, one can bring an uplifted appearance to sagging breasts. This toning process will also give maximum size to the smaller breasts and produce a lovelier appearance by encouraging good posture.

An easy, invigorating pepper-upper of the pectoral muscles has you standing upright, feet flat on the floor. Breathing deeply in and out, very slowly commence the crawl stroke, as in swimming. As one arm goes up, hand cupping out before you and ready to ascend and slowly sweep behind, the other arm begins its ascent. The only difference between this standing upright position and the actual swimming stroke is that you don't turn your head sideways any more than you have to. That is to say, do not hold the head rigid; allow it to turn a bit, but do not use the same head motion as in swimming.

Another breast developer has you in a standing position, lightly clasping your hands behind your back. Keeping the elbows stiff, very slowly raise the arms, at the same time slowly dipping the head and shoulders downward until the arms are directly overhead and the head and shoulders have dropped toward the knees. Keep the knees straight.

Start off slowly with this exercise, and do no more than two or three times a day for a week or more. Do not press beyond a point of comfort, nor force your arms upward into an uncomfortable position.

Another good exercise for toning the pectoral muscles and thereby giving better support to the breasts has you lying on the floor on your back, with your arms by your side. Take a deep breath and at the same time lift your arms upward and straight behind your head without bending your elbows. In the completed position, your body will be in one long line.

Without stopping the movement, return the arms to the sides of the body and back again. Repeat this movement ten times, for a week, then gradually work up to thirty movements each time.

BREAKFASTS FOR NOVEMBER

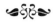

Cranberry juice
Sunflower eggs*
Herbal tea

Stewed prunes
Barley pancakes*
Herbal tea

Fresh blender applesauce
Granola (recipe on p. 21)
Herbal tea

Broiled banana
Oatmeal
Herbal tea

Grape juice
Wheat germ griddlecakes*
Herbal tea

Orange slices
Mushroom omelet
Herbal tea

Stewed apples
Millet cereal (recipe on p. 45)
Herbal tea

LUNCHES FOR NOVEMBER

Pumpkin soup*
Garbanzo salad*
Yogurt

Savory fish chowder*
Corn muffins
Yogurt

Chestnut soup*
Chinese cabbage salad
Yogurt

Cabbage soup
Nut fruit butter sandwiches
Yogurt

Vegetable soup
Cornmeal chapaties (recipe on p. 23)
Yogurt

Soybean soup
Green salad
Yogurt

Whole potato soup (recipe on p. 22)
Tomato omelet
Yogurt

DINNERS FOR NOVEMBER

Eggplant with cheese*
Rutabagas
Cabbage slaw

Liver patties*
Steamed parsleyed potatoes
Artichokes

Walnut and onion loaf*
Stewed tomatoes
Chinese cabbage

Chicken and brown rice
Spinach and onion salad

Broiled chicken livers
Eggplant
String beans

Lentil and rice stew*
Beets and onions
Sweet potatoes

Chop suey
Artichokes
Rice

RECIPES FOR NOVEMBER

Sunflower Eggs

2 beaten eggs
2 teaspoons ground sunflower
    seeds

sea salt
2 teaspoons water
1 tablespoon oil for scrambling

Beat together and scramble.

Barley Pancakes

2 tablespoons honey
½ cup warm water
1 cup barley flour
1 cup wheat germ

1 cup milk
2 beaten eggs
3 tablespoons salad oil

Mix the honey with the warm water and leave for 30 minutes. Add the flour, wheat germ, milk, eggs, and salad oil and beat well. Bake on a hot griddle.

Wheat Germ Griddlecakes

1 cup milk
½ cup brown rice flour
2 eggs with whites and yolks
    beaten separately

1 cup wheat germ
½ teaspoon sea salt

Add milk and flour to the beaten yolks. Blend in wheat germ and add salt, then fold in stiffly beaten egg whites. Bake on hot griddle.

Pumpkin Soup

2 cups raw, grated pumpkin	2 cups milk
2 cups chicken stock	2 tablespoons salad oil
1 tablespoon arrowroot	sea salt

Cook pumpkin in stock until soft. Mix arrowroot with enough milk to make a thin paste. Add remaining milk, oil, and salt to the first mixture and blend. Stir in the arrowroot paste and mix well. Pour into blender and reduce to a smooth consistency. Thin with additional milk if necessary.

Garbanzo Salad

1 cup garbanzo peas	¼ cup minced parsley
1 cup Chinese cabbage	2 leaves minced sweet basil
1 cup finely minced sweet onion	⅓ cup lemon juice
¼ cup minced sweet pepper	⅓ cup salad oil

Mix together and serve at room temperature.

Savory Fish Chowder

1 cup minced celery	2 teaspoons chervil
3 tablespoons salad oil	minced parsley
1½ cups cooked flaked fish (any firm-fleshed fish)	1 cup milk
½ cup chopped carrots	½ cup water
2 cups diced potatoes	sea salt

Sauté celery in oil until tender. Add carrots, potatoes, and water. Cover and cook until tender. Add remaining ingredients and cook until well heated.

Chestnut Soup

1 pound chestnuts　　　　　pinch mace
water　　　　　　　　　　　sea salt
2 pints chicken stock　　　2 cups milk
1 minced celery stalk　　　1 egg yolk

Drop the chestnuts into boiling water and allow to soak. Remove from pot. When the chestnuts are barely warm, remove the hulls and cook the nuts with the celery in the stock until both are soft. Add seasoning and strain the stock. Rub the chestnuts through a fine sieve, or place in blender with enough of the stock to make a smooth liquid. Mix some of the reserve stock with the beaten milk and egg yolk. Return to saucepan with remaining stock and heat. Thin with additional milk if too thick.

Eggplant with Cheese

1 minced onion　　　　　　½ teaspoon sweet basil
1 minced green pepper　　½ teaspoon oregano
½ cup salad oil　　　　　　sea salt
3 tomatoes　　　　　　　　cheese: any unprocessed
1 diced eggplant

Cook onion and pepper in oil until soft. Add tomatoes and eggplant, herbs, and salt to taste. Cover and cook until tender. Sprinkle ½ cup shredded cheese over the mixture, remove from heat, and cover for 5 minutes before serving.

Liver Patties

1 pound cooked liver	1 teaspoon savory
¼ cup wheat germ	2 beaten eggs
1 chopped onion	¾ teaspoon salt
2 tablespoons parsley	oil

Grind liver and the next four ingredients in a food grinder. Add the beaten eggs and salt and form into flat patties. Brush with oil and broil until done.

Walnut and Onion Loaf

1½ cups wheat germ	1 minced green pepper
½ cup cooked brown rice	1 minced celery stalk
milk	2 tablespoons salad oil
1 cup chopped walnuts	1 beaten egg
1 minced onion	2 tablespoons lemon juice

Soak wheat germ in enough milk to soften. Mix with remaining ingredients and bake in loaf pan until brown. Serve with tomato sauce.

Lentil and Rice Stew

1 cup lentils	1 cup diced carrots
4 cups chicken broth	1 diced turnip
1 cup brown rice	½ teaspoon marjoram
1 minced onion	sea salt

Cook lentils in 3 cups of the broth until tender. Add remaining broth and rice and cook until done. Stir in remaining vegetables, herbs, and salt and cook 15 to 20 minutes.

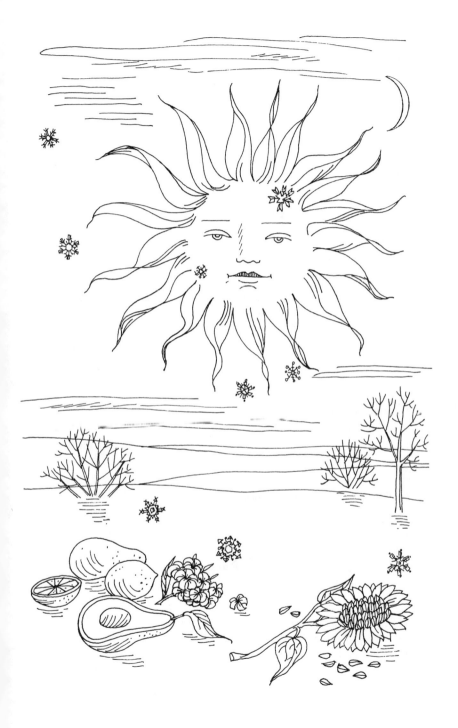

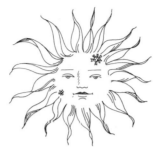

December

In the depths of drear December
When the white doth hide the green
Not a trembling weed up peereth
From its dark home underground.

                              Barry Cornwall

Originating from the Latin for "tenth month," which it was until
the calendar was changed, December now means cold, snow,
Christmas, winter sports, chafed skin, and days to go until next
year and a better life and a new you.

But who can call December drear when the jewel tones of
brilliant oranges, pale yellow grapefruits the color of a winter
sun and cheery red apples are offered us? In the warmer parts
of the world, nimble hands are reaching up for this wealth of
color and vitamins to ship to lands where not even a weed up-
peereth. In Florida, along the Rio Grande, in Israel, and in Spain,
lemons and limes fill baskets which head our way.

So eat your fruit and know it will put color into your wan
cheeks; know also that it will indeed be a better life if you start
now with your resolutions and spend this month exercising to get
into better shape by correcting figure faults and luxuriating in

things like a gelled milk bath and almond body lotion.

Oh, it is a busy month if you really care. Feed the skin, nourish the body, revitalize the hair, and reluctantly let go of the year, for you have learned so much and will be all the richer for your knowledge.

Did you know before now that the splendor of the oil-rich avocado can be made into a million-dollar facial, in addition to making a delicious salad which supplies the body with beauty vitamins and minerals? And look at the wealth you can carry into next year by regularly using an olive oil and herbal facial. Right in your own home you can prepare and use a wrinkle preventive which would cost a small fortune in a salon.

Pile into December and know that this is the last month and the last moments of a full and meaningful year, and that the manner in which you leave this month will determine your approach to the whole year ahead of you.

WINTER PORE REFINER

One of the biggest bugaboos of complexion care is enlarged pores. And this condition seems to become acute during the winter months when foods usually become heavier. Since we are not born with large pores, it seems that food habits may be one of their causes.

Fried foods have long been held responsible for bad skin. Greasy foods are hard to digest, and when the body cannot routinely dispose of wastes through conventional channels, it will use alternate routes. The skin can sometimes be imposed upon beyond its ability to cope with wastes. And it was never intended for greasy masses of impurities to pass through fine pore openings. But abuse of the body through improper diet can result in this.

Fresh fruits and vegetables used externally can sometimes help refine oversized pores. But this is December, so let's work with winter supplies.

Beat an egg white until it is firm, then add a small pinch (what you can hold between finger and thumb) of powdered camphor and continue beating until stiff. If powdered camphor is unobtainable, fold in a couple of drops of spirits of camphor.

Spread over the face in layers, adding a new layer when the first one dries. Leave on until the last layer dries, which should be thirty minutes or more. Rinse away with warm water, then dash cold water across the face and blot dry. Use this winter pore refiner at least twice a week for the best results. Avoid the area directly under the eyes, as this is a drying application.

GELLED MILK BATH

A silky-smooth bath water, laced with protein and fresh with herbal fragrances, helps tighten sagging skin and revive a winter-dried body. Instead of merely taking a bath, take a meaningful bath. Rushing through a tub of water does little for a body which needs help. Taking a moment to add some nutrition, serenity, or softener to your nightly tub can change your dreams to pleasure and restore your body at the same time.

These days our bodies are under assault from all kinds of pollution, which mixes with the body oils and clogs pores. At one time, a bath was taken for freshness, to cleanse the body of its own secretions. But today's environment demands the bath as a measure of safety from pollution and noxious gases in the atmosphere. Thus a bath with something extra is a necessity. Soap and water just aren't enough any more. They may cleanse the surface grime, but they won't restore. A restorative bath has some element of nutrition or other valuable ingredient in it. The gelled milk bath is a delight to take, and the body is cleansed and at the

same time protected with a thin film of nutritive ingredient.

Beat 1 whole egg until it is thick and lemon colored. Very slowly pour in 1 cup of herbal shampoo, and continue to beat as you pour. Sprinkle 1 tablespoon of unflavored gelatin into the mixture and continue to beat. Now add ½ cup of powdered skim milk and blend in well.

This will have to be stirred several times as it begins to set, or just before you scoop up a tablespoon or two for your bath each time. Hold a small handful (1 or 2 tablespoons) in your hand beneath the water faucet and allow the force of the falling water to homogenize it into your bathwater. No additional soap is needed with this bath.

AVOCADO FACIAL

The avocado is a vitamin- and mineral-rich food which should figure in the diet frequently, in addition to being used in complexion care. High in polyunsaturated oil, the avocado is an important beauty food, especially for those with dry skin. As a skin food, this vegetable with its impressive protein content offers nourishment to the complexion even as it softens and smooths wrinkles.

But it works best when mixed with lemon juice, so beat together a tablespoon of the ripest avocado and a few drops of real lemon juice. Blend together until you have a smooth paste. Apply to a freshly scrubbed face and throat. Leave on for 30 minutes and rinse away with warm, and then cool, water.

PEAR PEELER FACIAL

No matter what your skin type, chances are that in the month of December your complexion problems are intensified. Overheated houses, excessive carbohydrates in the diet, too little sunshine, and an atmosphere riddled with the waste from mass heating systems all tend to clog delicate skin openings and produce impacted pores which can't be cleaned with soap and water alone.

Frequent cleansing of the tissues is essential. And if you live in a large city, it is mandatory. But just any cleaning won't do. In the summertime, the soap and water routine may suffice, but winter weather and its attendant problems demand more heroic measures.

A little-known but effective skin peeler can be made from a ripe pear. It is true that it absorbs in a very moderate way, and takes only the dead top skin with it, but if it is used frequently enough, and as needed, then harsher methods aren't necessary.

Mash enough of a very ripe pear to create a tablespoon or so of the pulp. Massage gently into all areas of the face and neck, and allow to dry and remain on for an hour or more. Using a moistened beauty grain such as almond meal, rub across the covered area and then rinse away pear residue, flaking skin, and almond cleanser in warm water. Splash cool water onto the face and rub gently with a dry cloth to remove any last patches. Oil the face with a vegetable or nut oil, and blot dry.

OLIVE OIL AND HERB FACIAL
FOR WRINKLES

Women in Portugal, Spain, and Italy have incredibly fine complexions. And they also have one cosmetic item in common, virgin olive oil. Not only is the hair of these women unusually lustrous, but their skin remains supple and youthful long after women in other parts of the world have developed lines and creases which defy all known remedies.

If you are in your twenties, try an olive oil and herb pack as a preventive measure. Beyond that age, use this rewarding application to fight the encroachment of dry-skin wrinkles. Warm olive oil alone is helpful in softening harsh skin, but its benefits at least double when used in conjunction with various herbs.

Pour a small quantity of olive oil into a custard cup and heat over hot water until warm. Dip a cotton pad into the oil and rub into a freshly cleansed face (preferably cleansed with almond meal or oatmeal). Have another ceramic, glass, or stainless steel pot nearby with a tea made of dried nettle and dandelion leaves, from which set aside 1 cup to cool for a final pore-closing application.

For the herb infusion, drop a hearty handful of nettle and dandelion into 2 cups of boiling water, simmer for 3 or 4 minutes, and steep for 10.

Keep the liquid in the pot warm and dip a facecloth into it and apply to the face. If you don't want to lie down, you can hold it over your face until it cools. Dip into the tea solution and reapply at least five times.

Blot the skin dry and feel the fine texture that comes from this treatment.

SUNFLOWER MILK FOR CLEANSING

Supply any missing vitamin A and D in your complexion diet by cleansing your face with sunflower seed milk. This delicate wonder seed can be used to great advantage on distressed skins, especially those easily inflamed by surface irritations and rashes.

Vitamin D, difficult to obtain in plant form, is amply provided in sunflower seeds. Because of this flower's ability to swivel on its lengthy stalk as it follows the course of the sun from early morning until night, it totally absorbs ultraviolet rays, which help create vitamin D—much needed in December. Milk made from sunflower seeds both cleanses and tones the skin, leaving a fine softening film to nourish the starved tissues.

Grind ¼ cup of sunflower seeds. Add 1 cup of water and emulsify in the blender. Strain and use daily. Keep refrigerated. Or, better yet, drink the part you don't use on your face—double benefits this way. You might even learn to use this delicious milk on your cereals and so on. The results will eventually show themselves in a healthier complexion because of the calcium, in which many women are deficient, and vitamins A and D.

CREAMS FOR CHAPPED LIPS

To prevent lips from chafing, cracking, or peeling during the winter months, it is advisable to use a lip pomade or lipstick with healing waxes and oils in it. You don't see as many chapped lips today as you used to, mainly because of the increased use of lipstick with its protective covering. However, some lipsticks produce their own ills of bleeding and cracking if you are allergic to their ingredients.

If you cannot find a suitable lipstick, you might want to protect your lips from the raw winds which cause uncomfortable chafing of the lip area with a simply put together pomade.

Lip Pomade

Melt in a custard cup over low heat 2 ounces of white wax and 1 ounce of spermaceti. Beat in 2 ounces of raw honey and blend until well mixed. Slowly pour 4 ounces of sweet almond oil in a thin stream into the mixture, beating all the while. Remove from the heat and stir until the mixture is cool. Pour into a wide-mouthed jar for easy accessibility.

ALMOND MILK BODY LOTION

Just when you most need the protection of natural body oils, they seem to become the scarcest. Conditions of winter, whether from exposure or heated rooms, rob the body of the oils that keep the skin soft and resilient. Accumulating years can also bring about scant body oils. Neglected, roughened skin can develop into a chronic condition that is not only unattractive but is uncomfortable too, and can also lead to a myriad of troubles.

Almond milk lotion slides onto the body and brings with it vitamins A and B, calcium, phosphorus, potassium, and magnesium. The emollient properties of almonds make them an ideal cosmetic application for inflamed or dry, roughened skin. Two hundred years ago, practically every skin food, bleaching agent, hand cream, hair pomade, and beautifying product began with a sweet almond base, whether from almond oil or the crushed and sifted nut itself.

Blanch 1 ounce of almonds and remove the skins. Pat dry on paper toweling and put in a nut grinder or blender to reduce to a fine powder. Place the powder in the blender and add ½ pint of mineral water and homogenize. Strain the milky fluid through gauze and bottle for use after bathing. Rub over the entire body to soften and to feed dry and flaky skin.

DECEMBER COLORANT

Do you yearn for a summer's freshening breeze on your face? The warm flush from a radiant sun? They are, for many of us, far away in a southern climate. And here we are in frigid zones with drooping spirits and winter-fatigued complexions. But all is not lost. Just in time for the upcoming holidays, help is as near as a tidy mixture of whey, honey, and lemon juice.

Whey, which should be in everyone's pantry, and can be purchased in health food stores, is a milk product which aids the friendly bacteria to develop in the intestines and as such is quite an internal beauty-maker. (Whey is the clear liquid that separates from the curd when milk is curdled, as in making cream.) Used externally, whey can perk up a December wanness and cleanse a winter-embattled skin. Mix 1 teaspoon each of whey, lemon juice, and honey together. Spread across a clean face and allow to dry before rinsing off.

For super blood flushing of the skin, substitute apple cider vinegar for the lemon juice, avoiding the undereye area in both instances.

ROSE BUTTER FOR CHAFED HANDS

Don't for a moment let up on good hand care if you want to avoid the unpleasantness of drying skin and wrinkle clusters on the surface of the hands.

The most effective creams and lotions still seem to be the ones devised longer ago than anyone can remember, the ones that contain unusual foods rather than inert chemical ingredients. One comes across the highly praised preparations in ancient herbalists' books, family recipes, and, today, in natural cosmetic formulas.

The effectiveness of rose butter for distressed hands cannot be doubted, if only because its ingredients are so impressively good for you. Used singly, the ingredients can bring nutrition to dry, thirsty skin; used in combination, they will cause the fine skin on the backs of your hands to lose their taut look and raspy feel.

Allow ¼ pound (one stick) of *sweet* butter to soften at room temperature. Beat in 4 tablespoons of rose water, 2 beaten egg yolks, and 1 tablespoon of honey. When well mixed, beat into this enough finely powdered (use your blender) oatmeal to add firmness to the mixture.

Rub into the hands at night and rinse away in the morning with warm, and then cool, water and blot dry. Keep refrigerated, but allow the amount you will use each day to soften first.

WITCH HAZEL CREAM

Applications of simple, nourishing foods will usually take care of the most difficult of skins, relieve irritations, and safeguard the natural resiliency of the complexion. There are times, though, when some prefer a thick cosmetic cream for occasional use.

Witch hazel cream predates our own century. As a matter of fact, similar cold creams have been made for hundreds of years. The astringent witch hazel comes from a beautiful shrub growing in North America. According to the American Indians and the herbal lore they left behind, witch hazel has incredible healing powers. In any event, it is excellent as a bracing skin tonic and can be used to advantage as a skin toner.

Spermaceti is a waxy substance derived from the oil of the sperm whale. At one time, it was greatly used in cough medications. Now it is usually used in fine cosmetics, lotions, and soaps. We know the properties of sweet almond oil and its softening effects, plus the fact that lanolin is most nearly like the fat in the human body, and therefore easily absorbed by the human skin. Put all these ingredients together and you can produce a thick, creamy preparation which will soften and refine hardened skin.

Witch Hazel Cream

1 ounce spermaceti	1 dram tincture of benzoin
3 ounces sweet almond oil	3 ounces rose water
2 ounces lanolin	1 ounce witch hazel

Place the first three items in an enamel, glass, or stainless steel container over hot water. When the three ingredients have melted, remove from the heat and, beating all the while, allow to cool somewhat before adding 1 dram tincture of benzoin, 3 ounces of rose water (orange water, or mineral water), and 1 ounce of witch hazel. Beat until cold and pour into little jars.

ALMOND MEAL SHAMPOO

Want to give your hair a nutritious treatment with an unusual shampoo? One of the finest hair washes you can lavish on a scalp and hair which require extra attention is made from finely ground almond meal. This same food-turned-cosmetic serves admirably as a cleansing and luster-giving shampoo. As it cleanses, the almond meal adds its own fine oil and nutrients to create a silky head of hair in place of a dulled, robbed-of-life one.

Brush the hair thoroughly and then wet it in warm water. Use a small handful of almond meal at a time, and very carefully rub the meal into both hair and scalp. Add more water from time to time until a good lather forms from the meal. Massage the mixture not only into the scalp but throughout the hair strands, for this shampoo depends on being scoured through the hair for effectiveness.

Rinse under flowing warm water until all the grains are out and the water runs clear. This will take a bit longer than the usual shampoo, but can be easily done with a bit of patience and gives many rewards afterward. Use an apple cider vinegar or lemon juice final rinse by adding one or the other to the last water. Towel dry.

FRANGIPANI'S NIGHT GLOVES

The practice of using perfume began to spread across Europe with the return of the crusaders from the East. These fighters seemed to do as much conquering in the harems as they did on the battlefields, and the treasures within the harem won over more than a few. No doubt, these knights errant returned home with the exotic flower-oil scents that had enchanted them during their lusty forays, and they and their gifts found favor with the girls they left behind them.

As more and more adventuring took place, delightful scents from all corners of the world were discovered, and to women, a botanist on Christopher Columbus' ship might have played as important a role as Columbus' chief navigator if he turned up another perfumed plant or bit of spice which could be used to anoint them.

Mercutio Frangipani, a botanist who set sail with Columbus on his voyage to America, discovered, in Antigua, a sweet-smelling plant which was later given his name. His descendant, the Marquis de Frangipani, proceeded to create a perfume of exquisite scent from this flower, and to use it in a pomade which he lathered into his gloves.

From these gloves evolved the idea of an easy, all-in-one operation to soften and restore needed moisture and oils to parched, roughened hands, at the same time leaving a healing film over them and scenting them.

Honey and almond paste is worn at night under kid gloves at least three sizes too large. This is the same formula used a century ago, and it is just as effective and just as much needed today for the woman who wants beautiful hands and knows that she must work for them especially after using a few bars of the usual soap and washing dishes with skin-destroying detergents.

Frangipani's Night Gloves

8 ounces raw honey	½ ounce egg yolk
4 ounces almond meal	8 ounces sweet almond oil

Heat the honey over water to an easy-flowing consistency. Pour into the almond meal and knead it together with the well-beaten egg yolk. Add the almond oil and knead until a smooth paste is formed.

Rub thoroughly into clean hands just before retiring and pull on oversize kid gloves. Keep the paste in the refrigerator and remove enough to use at one time to warm at room temperature well ahead of bedtime.

APHRODISIAC FOR DECEMBER

The warming qualities of love are especially appreciated during this cold month. We need a bright spot in our lives when all else is dull and dreary. To cheer ourselves—and to be able to stimulate others—it's good to exert a little extra effort in winter, when we can so easily be dragged down. Unfortunately, far too many women are literally too exhausted to be interested in this lovely part of living. Many times their fatigue and indifference can be traced to an iron deficiency.

Every cell in the body contains a certain amount of iron, and the body must be fed a steady supply of this vital metal in order to maintain the production of red blood cells. When an iron deficiency occurs, ills develop, too, including strawlike hair, gray complexions, and premature aging. Iron deficiency also results in a loss of energy and vitality, which in turn produces an unresponsive person.

Be wise and add iron-rich foods to your daily diet. Use barley, peanut and soybean flours, liver, wheat germ, parsley, dandelion greens, and dried fruits.

And why not be charming about it and ensure your response to an amorous evening by adding apricots, a good source of iron, to your menu? Mix 1 cup of stewed apricots with ½ cup of freshly grated coconut and 2 teaspoons of grated lemon peel. Serve with custard sauce or cream.

ANKLE AND FOOT EXERCISES

The prettiest rose would not be so lovely if it sat upon a thickened branch instead of its own delicate stem. And the most attractive leg requires a slender ankle to complete the picture. Ankles which have been allowed to develop excess flesh and fat can be rather easily restored to the correct proportions if enough time and attention are given them. And ankle exercises can be done at odd moments, even when you are seated.

An alternate rolling outward and inward from the soles of the feet gets at puffy ankle fat from all angles and helps to trim it away. Stand upright and stockingless, with your feet a foot apart. Roll them out as far as comfortably possible and then slowly roll them inward. Continue this rotating movement several times. Gradually work up to two or three minutes a day.

Though crossed legs are never attractive and restrict blood flow through the veins, the following exercise requires a brief crossing. But since it is only for a short time and the full weight of the leg never rests on the thigh during the movements, don't worry. Cross the left leg over the right, clearing the right knee. Rotate the left foot in a complete circle ten times forward. Reverse to the left and repeat. Do the same exercise with the right foot both forward and in reverse.

Stimulation and fat reduction in the ankle area can be accomplished during odd moments. Before sitting down at your desk, you could give a few minutes to this usually neglected area. Shuck your shoes and hold on to the chair back. Extend your right leg before you with the toes touching the floor. Tense the leg and slowly pull your foot along the floor toward you, dropping the ball of the foot and then the heel until the foot is flat as it glides under your back to rise onto the toes as it extends to the rear. Drop the foot flat then raise the toes upward and slide it back under your body on the heel to the front position. Once again point the toes and repeat. Repeat with the left leg.

BREAKFASTS FOR DECEMBER

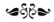

Mixed fresh grapefruit and orange slices
Carrot pancakes*
Herbal tea

Stewed dried apricots
Baked breakfast rice
Herbal tea

Fresh applesauce
Eggs fines herbes
Whole grain muffins
Herbal tea

Stewed prunes and lemons
Oatmeal
Herbal tea

Broiled apple slices
Cornmeal mush and maple syrup
Herbal tea

Fresh orange
Barley pancakes (recipe on p. 262)
Herbal tea

LUNCHES FOR DECEMBER

᠊ᢀᠼᢀ᠊

Egg Foo Yung with sprouts (recipe on p. 214)
Whole grain bread
Yogurt

Soybean soup
Vegetable sticks
Yogurt

Chestnut soup (recipe on p. 264)
Green salad sprinkled with sunflower meal
Yogurt

Cottage cheese and shredded vegetables
Stuffed eggs
Yogurt

Lentil soup
Cheese and apples
Yogurt

Vegetable soup
Avocado slices with banana and grapefruit
Yogurt

Cream of mushroom soup
Shredded cabbage, green pepper, radishes, and celery
Yogurt

DINNERS FOR DECEMBER

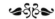

Sautéed brain slices
Mashed rutabagas
Coleslaw

Eggplant patties*
Stuffed tomatoes
Brussels sprouts

Baked potatoes stuffed with cheese
Broccoli
Mushrooms stuffed with nuts

Banana slices with chicken livers en brochette
Brown rice cooked in broth
String beans

Sardines with lemon juice and chopped green onions
Cauliflower
Sautéed mung sprouts

Broiled kidney
Baked sweet potatoes
Steamed onions and sprouts

Broiled sweetbreads
Parsleyed potatoes in skin
Chopped steamed beet tops

RECIPES FOR DECEMBER

Carrot Pancakes

1 shredded carrot
1 shredded potato
1 minced onion
2 tablespoons wheat germ

1 tablespoon arrowroot
1 teaspoon chervil
sea salt

Place one vegetable at a time in blender to reduce to finest pulp. Remove and add remaining ingredients. Sauté in vegetable oil over low heat and brown.

Eggplant Patties

1 chopped eggplant
2 cups ground sunflower meal
½ cup wheat germ
1 minced onion

1 teaspoon savory
2 beaten eggs
1 tablespoon vegetable oil
sea salt

Peel and cook eggplant in a small amount of water until tender. Mix the next seven ingredients together and blend in the eggplant. Make into little cakes and sauté in a lightly oiled skillet until brown.

Sources of Supply for Natural Beauty Products

Vegetable, nut, and fruit oils are available in health food shops and from mail-order natural food houses. They also stock all natural foods such as oats, barley, brewer's yeast, and whole grain flours, in addition to sea salt, natural vitamins, herbal teas, seeds to sprout, nuts, and yogurt. Many of these products are also carried in supermarkets which have health food sections.

Most pharmacies carry the following supplies or can special order them on request: benzoin, camphor, cocoa butter, complexion brushes, beeswax, ethyl alcohol, Fuller's earth, gum arabic, hydrous lanolin, perfumed oils, unscented talcum, witch hazel, and essential oils.

Other sources which will send a catalogue upon request include:

Indiana Botanic Gardens, Inc.
Hammond, Indiana 46325

Caswell-Massey Co., Ltd.
114 East 25th Street
New York, New York 10010

Nature's Herb Company
281 Ellis Street
San Francisco, California 94102

Haussmann's Pharmacy
6th and Girard Avenue
Philadelphia, Pennsylvania 19123

Comfrey plants can be obtained from:

North Central Comfrey Producers
Box 195B
Glidden, Wisconsin 54527

Potpourri, dried, can be obtained from:

Caprilands Herb Farm
Silver Street
Coventry, Connecticut 06238

All ingredients mentioned in this book should be available from one of these sources.

Index

73 74 75 76 77 10 9 8 7 6 5 4 3 2 1